Gendered Violence, Mental Health and Recovery in Everyday Lives

W0113837

Gendered Violence, Mental Health and Recovery in Everyday Lives: Beyond Trauma offers new insights into the social dimensions of emotional distress in abuse-related mental health problems, and explores the many interconnections between gendered violence, different forms of abuse and poor mental health. Looking at how individuals can overcome the impact of abuse over the course of their lives, Moulding maps a feminist-informed, recovery-oriented approach to therapy and prevention.

Drawing on sociological perspectives and a wide range of international research, as well as original qualitative data presented here for the first time, this book:

- Demonstrates how gender and other social power relations play out in the specific emotional dimensions of some of the mental health problems most strongly linked to abuse, including post-traumatic stress disorder, anxiety, depression and eating disorders.
- Critiques the way that mainstream psychological theory and research pathologises the effects of abuse through various mental illness diagnoses, obscuring the nature of the individual emotional distress involved, its social context and relational nature.
- Outlines a feminist-informed, recovery-oriented approach that aims to reduce violence against women and children.

This innovative volume is an important contribution to the literature on the impact of violence and abuse on the lives and health of its survivors. It will be of interest to students and researchers from a range of disciplines and professions, including social work, gender studies, sociology, social policy, psychology, counselling, mental health, public health, medicine and nursing.

Nicole Moulding is Senior Lecturer at the University of South Australia, Australia. A qualified social worker, her teaching and research interests are in the areas of gender and mental health, gendered violence and abuse, and interpretive research methodologies.

Routledge studies in the sociology of health and illness

Gendered Violence, Mental Health and Recovery in Everyday Lives
Beyond trauma
Nicole Moulding

Forthcoming titles:

Vaginal Examination in Labour
Challenging contemporary practice
Mary Stewart

Bodily Exchanges, Bioethics and Border Crossing
Perspectives on giving, selling and sharing bodies
Edited by Erik Malmqvist and Kristin Zeiler

Transnationalising Reproduction
Third party conception in a globalised world
Edited by Roisin Ryan Flood and Jenny Gunnarsson Payne

Gendered Violence, Mental Health and Recovery in Everyday Lives

Beyond trauma

Nicole Moulding

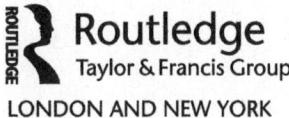
Routledge
Taylor & Francis Group

LONDON AND NEW YORK

First published 2016
by Routledge
4 Park Square, Milton Park, Abingdon, Oxon OX14 4RN
605 Third Avenue, New York, NY 10017

First issued in paperback 2023

Routledge is an imprint of the Taylor & Francis Group, an informa business

British Library Cataloguing-in-Publication Data
A catalogue record for this book is available from the British Library

Library of Congress Cataloging in Publication Data
Moulding, Nicole, author.
Gendered abuse, violence and mental health in everyday lives : beyond
trauma / Nicole Moulding.
    p. ; cm.
    Includes bibliographical references and index.
    I. Title.
    [DNLM: 1. Adult Survivors of Child Abuse–psychology. 2. Domestic
    Violence–psychology. 3. Mental Health. 4. Women–psychology. WM 167]
    RC569.5.C55
    616.85′822390651–dc23   2015019878

ISBN: 978-0-415-73945-0 (hbk)
ISBN: 978-1-315-81663-0 (ebk)
ISBN: 978-0-367-34580-8 (pbk)

DOI: 10.4324/9781315816630

Typeset in Times New Roman
by Wearset Ltd, Boldon, Tyne and Wear

Publisher's Note
The publisher has gone to great lengths to ensure the quality of this reprint but
points out that some imperfections in the original copies may be apparent.

This book is dedicated to Matthew, Sophie and Jack.
Your support and understanding has made it possible.

Contents

Acknowledgements

First of all, I would like to thank all those individuals who participated in the research that forms the basis of this book. The generous giving of your time to help increase understanding about gendered violence, abuse and mental health has been greatly appreciated. Next, I would like to acknowledge and thank my colleagues. I am fortunate indeed to work with many wonderful women whose conversation, thoughts and critical insights have been crucially important to me in drawing this work together. Thanks go to Sarah Wendt, Fiona Buchanan, Suzanne Franzway, Carole Zufferey, Donna Chung, Alison Elder and Deirdre Tedmanson. Also, additional thanks to Alison Elder for helping out with some of the administrative tasks.

1 Introduction

An interconnected approach

Male-perpetrated violence and abuse against women and girls is a major social and public health problem across the globe (World Health Organization (WHO), 2013), and helping professionals come across it regularly in their day-to-day work. In addition to responding at the point of crisis, they will also see many women struggling down the track with emotional distress. However, while the idea that gendered violence and abuse is linked to later mental health problems is now widely accepted, this has not always been the case. Attention to the impact of male-perpetrated violence and abuse on women's mental health has ebbed and flowed along with cyclic 're-discoveries' of child sexual abuse, and with waves of concern and indifference about domestic violence and sexual assault. We seem to be going through a period of re-discovery of gendered violence and its effects at the moment with enquiries into institutionalised child sexual, physical and emotional abuse and regular media reports of domestic violence in Australia and elsewhere. While increased attention to gendered violence and abuse, and its negative impact on women, might provide opportunities for change, there are also risks associated with such a re-discovery, including the further promulgation of the 'harm' story of abuse (O'Dell, 2003), which assumes that gendered violence and abuse invariably result in psychological problems for women. At this point in time, psychological trauma models of the effects of gendered violence and abuse represent the dominant 'harm' story.

This book is not about revealing the 'truth' of gendered violence and abuse, and their impact on emotional wellbeing: there are many competing truths with their own contradictory evidence bases. Rather, what this book seeks to do is explore and examine gendered violence and mental health in an interconnected way, and at a number of different levels. A robust body of feminist research and scholarship already exists in this area, and has examined the impact of child sexual abuse (O'Dell, 2003; Warner and Wilkins, 2003; Warner, 2009) and domestic violence (Humphreys and Thiara, 2003; Laing and Toivonen, 2010; Laing, Irwin and Toivonen, 2010) on women's mental health. This book builds on this work and seeks to be distinctive in two main ways. First, it considers the impact of a range of different types of gendered violence and abuse on women's mental health, particularly childhood emotional abuse, childhood sexual abuse and domestic violence. Different types of abuse often occur together (Fleming et al., 1999;

Humphreys and Thiara, 2003), and are known to have more negative effects when they do (Messman-Moore and Garrigus, 2007). More significantly, though, considering the diversity of gendered violence and abuse on women's mental health acknowledges that similar systems of social meaning and gender power relations based on male privilege frame all types of gendered violence and abuse: as such, there are likely to be some commonalities in women's understandings and experiences of mental health problems in contexts of violence and abuse. This is not to suggest that women's experiences are the same, because they clearly are not, situated as they are within diverse power relations including those of class, race and sexuality, and I also attend to these in addition to gender relations.

The second point of difference is that this book seeks to engage with women's understandings and experiences of gendered violence, abuse and mental health at a number of levels. Existing feminist research in this area tends to be either post-structural or materialist and structural feminist. The former tradition includes feminist scholarship into child sexual abuse and mental health (O'Dell, 2003; Warner, 2009) while the latter includes feminist attention to domestic violence and mental health (Humphreys and Thiara, 2003; Laing and Toivonen, 2010). As such, feminist work on child sexual abuse considers how gendered social discourses frame women's understandings and experiences and takes a critical approach to the dominance of pathologising psycho-medical discourses in this area. The more materialist approaches to domestic violence and mental health tend to centre unequal gender and other social power relations and women's own voices of their lived experiences. These different emphases to some extent reflect the different disciplinary backgrounds of the respective researchers, with many of the feminists who focus on child sexual abuse emanating from critical psychology, while feminists researching domestic violence often hail from social work, as I do myself. In the three research studies that represent the basis for most of this book, I attempt to navigate both the discursive and the material dimensions of women's understandings and experiences of gendered violence, abuse and mental health. In order to do this, I adopt McNay's (2004) concept of situated intersubjectivity, which understands the discursive aspects of identity and everyday intersubjective material power relations as inherently intertwined. McNay (2004) argues that the concept of situated intersubjectivity is a useful corrective to the individualising tendencies of post-structuralism because it explicitly embeds the subject in social relations, but also counteracts a materialist tendency to prioritise structures over experience by emphasising intention and agency on the part of the subject. Situated intersubjectivity is therefore a useful theoretical frame for researching women's understandings and experiences of emotional distress in the context of violent and abusive social relations of gender because it enables attention to social discourses, women's agency, the material impact of abuse on women's bodies and emotions, and the structural power relations these are embedded within. However, attending to these different threads simultaneously is not straightforward, and I consider some of the challenges associated with this in the following chapters.

Taking a gender perspective

Child sexual abuse and domestic violence are widely understood to be gendered experiences because women and girls are so disproportionately affected, and males are overwhelmingly the perpetrators. Thus, it is hardly radical to assert that these problems are gendered. However, to include childhood emotional abuse as a gendered form of abuse is more unusual. My interests in childhood emotional abuse initially arose from work as a feminist social worker in women's health. More recent emerging quantitative evidence reveals that childhood emotional abuse is the most common form of child abuse (Australian Institute of Health and Welfare (AIHW), 2014; Stoltenborgh, 2012) and it is increasingly linked by researchers to poor mental health (O'Dougherty Wright *et al.*, 2009), even more strongly than for other forms of abuse (Schneider *et al.*, 2007; O'Dougherty Wright *et al.*, 2009). There is also some evidence that childhood emotional abuse is more commonly reported by women and girls (Cawson *et al.*, 2000; Scher *et al.*, 2004). However, understanding the gendered dimensions of non-sexual forms of abuse needs to extend beyond counts of who is abusing who to situate the phenomenon in its wider gendered social context (May-Chahal, 2006). The feminist research presented in this book on childhood emotional abuse therefore represents the first attempt to examine how gender discourses, practices and power relations frame this type of abuse.

I need to point out, though, that none of the research undertaken for this book is concerned with contributing to evidence about the causative links between abuse and particular categories of mental illness: the research presented here is qualitative and therefore cannot, and does not seek to, prove or disprove causation. Moreover, while the question of causation remains contested and even controversial for some, strong associations between gendered violence, abuse and mental health problems have already been demonstrated through quantitative research. On the basis of this, it has been estimated that childhood sexual abuse increases an individual's risk of common mental health problems by as much as four times (Briere and Elliot, 1994). This does not mean that all people with mental health problems have been abused or that all people who are abused will experience mental health problems. Nor does it mean that abuse is the only 'causative factor' for mental health problems in individuals who have experienced abuse. What it does mean is that abuse substantially increases a person's chances of experiencing mental health problems. Rather than causation, what this book is concerned with is how experiences of gendered violence and abuse are understood, lived and responded to. Mental health problems continue to be predominantly explained through medical and psychological theories and practices that pathologise the abused individual (and the perpetrator, too) as damaged and dysfunctional, largely ignoring the social contexts of abuse. Instead, this book explores the social dimensions of gendered violence and abuse, and its impact on emotional wellbeing. This includes how social power relations not only help to determine who gets abused, how and by who, but how these relations become deeply inscribed in the specific emotional and psychological dimensions of mental illnesses. Thus, I locate mental illness and its emotional distress in social relationships (Tew, 2008) rather than inside individuals alone, and therefore in the discourses, power relations and practices that structure these relationships.

Situating myself in feminism

During my social work studies in the early 1980s, along with many of my fellow students, I discovered feminism. For me, feminism was the foundational knowledge that enabled the naming of gender power relations and the difficulties experienced by women that seemed to flow from them. My honours-level thesis was on domestic violence and I went on to work as a social worker in women's health and then community health. I became particularly interested in gender and mental health during this period, struck by how commonly experiences of gendered violence and abuse appeared as the backdrop to women's struggles with anxiety, depression, eating disorders and more general feelings of low self-worth. When I came to do a PhD, I chose to focus on eating disorders because they seemed to demonstrate particularly well how gender discourses and practices can play out in so-called mental illness. I was especially fascinated by how psychiatry continued to reproduce pathologising, individualistic understandings and paternalistic treatments in spite of evidence that their approaches were out of step with women's lived experiences and more often than not failed to bring about recovery (Moulding, 2003, 2006). However, as my research in this area progressed, I became increasingly aware of the spectre of violence and abuse once again in the backgrounds of many (not all) of the women I interviewed. And so I found that I had come full circle in confronting the impact of violence and abuse in women's lives. However, feminist theorising, research and practice had changed enormously since the 1980s. While earlier feminist scholarship into both gendered violence and mental health was materialist and structuralist, post-structural feminism has enabled us to ask different questions and gain new insights into the complexities of gender discourses and mental health without losing sight of the social structures of male privilege in which women and children live. More recently, many feminists are now grappling with the challenge of uniting concerns over the discursive dimensions of women's experience with their basis in material, structural gender power relations of male privilege (see McNay, 2004), and this book attempts to take up this challenge.

Outline of the book

The book is based on three research studies into gendered violence, abuse and mental health. In Chapter 2, I map existing understandings of the links between abuse and mental illness in the psycho-medical literature and contrast this with feminist research and scholarship on gendered violence, abuse and mental health. In Chapter 3, I explain further my theoretical and methodological approach to undertaking research into gendered violence, abuse and mental health, elaborating the feminist theoretical frame adopted for this research and outlining the methods used for the three studies. The subsequent chapters then present and discuss key findings from the three studies.

In the first study, which is presented in Chapter 4, I focus on childhood emotional abuse because, as noted earlier, it has not been studied by feminist scholars but has been linked the most strongly with mental health problems. This study therefore asked how gender (and race and class) frames childhood emotional abuse and, in turn, how it frames the subsequent mental health problems experienced by individuals.

For the second study, presented in Chapter 5, I focused on eating disorders as illustrative of a mental health problem that is not only strongly associated with abuse but is overwhelmingly diagnosed in women rather than men. Women diagnosed with eating disorders have been deeply pathologised in highly gendered ways within psycho-medicine (Moulding, 2003, 2006) and this study asked how experiences of violence and abuse might play out in the particular symptomologies associated with these conditions, and the social contexts and social meanings framing this.

Chapter 6 explores women's narratives and experiences of mental health problems in response to domestic violence. The chapter examines how women construct the impact of domestic violence on their sense of themselves, their identities and emotions, and critically explores medical and psychological discourses commonly used in this area. In different ways, Chapters 4, 5 and 6 demonstrate how women's emotional distress in response to gendered violence and abuse is framed by gendered discourses that involve fundamental contradictions about femininity and selfhood, which are also reproduced in the dominant psycho-medical discourses applied to understanding women's mental health. Chapter 7 then considers the scope for feminist-informed intervention, both in terms of therapeutic interventions and prevention.

The development of appropriate responses to mental health problems in contexts of violence and abuse first involves taking a critical perspective on received wisdoms about how these experiences have been understood. The following chapter specifically explores the role of psycho-medical theory and research in individualising and pathologising mental health problems in contexts of abuse, followed by attention to feminist approaches that bring new understandings of women's experiences beyond the narrow view of mainstream research.

References

Australian Institute of Health and Welfare (AIHW) (2014) *Child Protection Australia 2012–2013*. Canberra: Australian Government. Available at: www.aihw.gov.au/publication-detail/?id=60129547965, accessed 22 April 2015.

Briere, J. and Elliot, D.M. (1994) Immediate and long-term impacts of child sexual abuse, *The Future of Children: Sexual Abuse of Children*, 4(2), pp. 54–69.

Cawson, P., Wattam, C., Brooker, C. and Kelly, G. (2000) *Child Maltreatment in the United Kingdom: A Study of the Prevalence of Child Abuse and Neglect*. London: NSPCC.

Fleming, J., Mullen, P.E., Sibthorne, B. and Gammer, G. (1999) The long-term impact of child sexual abuse in Australian women, *Child Abuse & Neglect*, 23(2), pp. 145–159.

Humphreys, C. and Thiara, R. (2003) Mental health and domestic violence: 'I call it symptoms of abuse', *British Journal of Social Work*, 33(2), pp. 209–226.

Laing, L. and Toivonen, C. (2010) *Evaluation of the Domestic Violence and Mental Health Pilot Project*. Faculty of Education and Social Work, University of Sydney.

Laing, L., Irwin, J. and Toivonen, C. (2010) Women's stories of collaboration between domestic violence and mental health services, *Communities, Children and Families Australia*, 5 (2), pp. 18–30.

McNay, L. (2004) Situated intersubjectivity. In B. Marshall and A. Witz (eds), *Engendering the Social: Feminist Encounters with Sociological Theory*. Maidenhead: Open University Press, pp. 171–186.

May-Chahal, C. (2006) Gender and child maltreatment: the evidence base, *Social Work and Society*, 4(1), pp. 53–68.

Messman-Moore, T.L. and Garrigus, A.S. (2007) The association of child abuse and eating disorder symptomatology: the importance of multiple forms of abuse and re-victimization, *Journal of Aggression, Maltreatment & Trauma*, 14(3), pp. 51–72.

Moulding, N.T. (2003) Constructing the self in mental health practice: identity, individualism and the feminisation of deficiency, *Feminist Review*, 75, pp. 57–74.

Moulding, N.T. (2006) Disciplining the feminine: the reproduction of gender contradictions in the mental health care of women with eating disorders, *Social Science & Medicine*, 62(4), pp. 793–804.

O'Dell, L. (2003) The 'harm' story in child sexual abuse: contested understandings, disputed knowledges. In P. Reavey and S. Warner (eds), *New Feminist Stories of Child Sexual Abuse: Sexual Scripts and Dangerous Dialogues*. London: Routledge, pp. 131–147.

O'Dougherty Wright, M., Crawford, E. and Del Castillo, D. (2009) Childhood emotional maltreatment and later psychological distress among college students: the mediating role of maladaptive schemas, *Child Abuse and Neglect*, 33, pp. 59–68.

Scher, C.D., Forde, D.R., McQuaid, J.R. and Stein, M.B. (2004) Prevalence and demographic correlates of childhood maltreatment in an adult community sample, *Child Abuse and Neglect*, 28(2), pp. 167–180.

Schneider, R., Baumrind, N. and Kimerling, R. (2007) Exposure to child abuse and risk for mental health problems in women, *Violence and Victims*, 22(5), pp. 620–631.

Stoltenborgh, M. (2012) The universality of childhood emotional abuse: a meta-analysis of worldwide prevalence, *Journal of Aggression, Maltreatment and Trauma*, 21(8), pp. 870–890.

Tew, Jerry (2008) Social perspectives on mental distress. In T. Stickley and T. Basset (eds), *Learning about Mental Health Practice*. Chichester: John Wiley & Sons Ltd, pp. 235–252.

Warner, S. (2009) *Understanding the Effects of Child Sexual Abuse: Feminist Revolutions in Theory, Research and Practice*. London: Routledge.

Warner, S. and Wilkins, T. (2003) Diagnosing distress and reproducing disorder: women, child sexual abuse and 'borderline personality disorder'. In P. Reavey and S. Warner (eds), *New Feminist Stories of Child Sexual Abuse: Sexual Scripts and Dangerous Dialogues*. London: Routledge, pp. 167–186.

World Health Organization (WHO) (2013) *Global and Regional Estimates of Violence against Women: Prevalence and Health Effects of Intimate Partner Violence and Non-Partner Sexual Violence*. Geneva: WHO. Available at: www.who.int/reproductive-health/publications/violence/9789241564625/en/, accessed 22 April 2015.

2 Putting gender in the frame

The recognition of gendered violence and abuse as social problems has been relatively recent, triggered in large part by the second wave feminist movement and emerging stories of women's experiences of domestic violence, rape and child sexual abuse. This recognition, in turn, has led to a burgeoning of research over the past four decades, with a significant amount of attention directed to the effects of violence and abuse on women's mental health. Feminist scholars and helping professionals have been instrumental in drawing attention to gendered violence and abuse, and its negative impact on emotional wellbeing, and continue to provide services and support in this area, however mainstream psychology and medicine have become increasingly prominent in this field. Moreover, while there was initially a level of exchange between feminism and the helping professions on the subject of gendered violence and its effects, the direction of this has become increasingly one-directional with many feminist practitioners now drawing on psychological concepts such as 'trauma' but arguably few mainstream practitioners drawing on feminist understandings of gendered violence and abuse. This chapter critically explores historical and contemporary knowledge about gender violence, abuse and their impact on emotional wellbeing as the backdrop to positioning the feminist research that forms the basis of the following chapters.

Ebbs and flows: the emergence of gendered violence and abuse as social problems

Male-perpetrated violence against women and children has not always been recognised as such. It was primarily during the Enlightenment in the eighteenth and nineteenth centuries that social reformers in English-speaking countries such as Australia, the United Kingdom and United States began to target domestic violence and child abuse as problematic and therefore as requiring intervention. As noted by Stark (2007), domestic violence went largely unremarked and was accepted as simply part of life prior to this, unless it took the extreme form of 'wife torture' or murder (p. 143). The prohibition of violence against wives occurred first in the United States in 1641, however, little action was taken until the mid-nineteenth century when the women's temperance movement made links between wife beating, divorce and women's suffrage and many states outlawed or limited the legal right of men to beat their wives (Stark, 2007). In the UK, the women's movement was more directly involved in legislative efforts to outlaw domestic violence, and a man's right to 'chastisement' of his wife was abolished in 1829 and wife beating was outlawed in 1853 (Stark, 2007). Feminist campaigners such as Frances Cobbe argued that domestic violence persisted because men saw women as property and she and other feminist reformers demanded full economic and social justice for women, however, domestic violence continued to be understood as a problem of the poorer classes, immigrants and blacks (Stark, 2007).

In reference to child abuse and neglect, concern about the treatment of children also emerged in the eighteenth and nineteenth centuries, motivated in part by the shift to the state in managing its resources in the form of healthy labouring bodies, including those of children (Bell, 2011). Not dissimilarly to wives, children were the legal property of their fathers prior to this. Foucault notes that in ancient times, 'the ancient patria potestas ... granted the father of the Roman family the right to dispose of the life of his children and his slaves: just as he had given them life, so he could take it away' (Foucault, 1990, cited in Bell, 2011: 101). The eighteenth and nineteenth centuries therefore saw the 'birth of childhood', the preserve of upper-class children initially but later extended to children more generally (Bell, 2011). Alongside the idea of childhood came notions of children's innocence, dependency and need for guidance and discipline, with the family increasingly understood as the unit that develops children's bodies as healthy labourers (Bell, 2011). In this context, child maltreatment and neglect came to be seen as detrimental to such ends and therefore as necessitating intervention. The rise of 'child saver movements' in the United States and United Kingdom in the nineteenth and twentieth centuries further established child abuse as a social problem and intervention as the responsibility of the state (Costin *et al.*, 1996) leading to early practices of removing poor urban children into institutions (Bell, 2011). The emergence of the professional social worker in the early 1900s and their role in child protection also helped make child abuse more visible (Hacking, 1988). However, up until the 1970s, child abuse continued to primarily refer to physical abuse and neglect (Hacking, 1988), and while both fathers and mothers could be held responsible, there was a greater focus on mothers and little attention to the psychological impact on children beyond the risk of 'delinquency'.

Acknowledgement of child sexual abuse has had a far rockier road to acknowledgement and intervention. Sexual relations between adults and children have been documented from ancient times, but were not necessarily framed as problematic or abusive. The specific 'discovery' of sexual abuse by Sigmund Freud in the late nineteenth century marks an important point in the ebb and flow of recognition in the modern era. Freud's theory of the role of sexual abuse in hysteria and his subsequent retraction have been covered in some detail by other authors and will only be described briefly here (for a fuller account, see Breckenridge, 1999). In short, Freud asserted that many of the symptoms of so-called hysteria in his female patients reflected underlying traumatic experiences of sexual abuse in the family at the hands of male relatives, including fathers, and he documented his observations in his paper 'The aetiology of hysteria', presented in 1896 (Breckenridge, 1999). Freud's claims were met, first, with silence, then with disbelief and then with censure by his colleagues (Breckenridge, 1999). He recanted his view by instead arguing, in what Breckenridge (1999) calls an 'astonishing turnaround', that his patients' stories of sexual abuse were 'seduction fantasies' (p. 17). Freud then went on to formulate his much better received psychoanalytic theory of the Oedipal Complex, and children (especially girls) became not the victims of sexual abuse but blamed for sexual trauma instead through the notion of the 'seductive child' (Breckenridge, 1999). As is pointed out by Breckenridge (1999), this history has had two main related repercussions that have rolled on down through the ages: first, victims' voices have been silenced and, second, child sexual abuse came to be spoken about in mythologised terms rather than as a real, lived experience.

There was some muted professional recognition of child sexual abuse in first half of the twentieth century after Freud's retraction. Levett (2003) notes that, in the wake of the Second World War, there was a rise in 'victimology' as a result of moves to increase professionalisation and develop social policies to redress the problems of various groups in Western societies. She argues that the contemporary preoccupation with the damaging effects of child sexual abuse grew hand-in-hand with the modern emergence of the professions of medicine and law as social institutions (Levett, 2003). In relation to incest, there was a dominant view in the 1950s that sexual abuse occurred only within dysfunctional families, and that women were largely responsible because they had failed in their roles as wives and mothers, for example, in being sexually unavailable or insufficiently caring (Laing, 1999). Men who sexually abused their own children were understood as troubled and the sexual motivation of their offending was played down, unlike for extra-familial sex offenders (Laing, 1999). The middle of the twentieth century therefore saw a more general retreat from recognition and action in response to gendered violence and abuse and a growing emphasis on mother-blame, even among those groups who had been active in reform previously. Thus, while early reformers saw domestic violence, child abuse and child sexual abuse as originating in illegitimate male power in the home, and there were some efforts by police to remove offenders and safeguard women and children, these same groups came to see divorce, female employment and suffrage as a threat to domestic harmony (Stark, 2007). This led to a preoccupation with 'female correction' in cases of domestic violence and child abuse, cementing a woman- and mother-blame approach that has characterised much of family services ever since (Jones, 1998; Stark, 2007).

Not dissimilarly to the fields of domestic violence and child protection, the focus of psychology and psychiatry more generally during this period was on the role of mothers in damaging their children. Horsfall (1991) argues that the patriarchal nature of psychiatry has made it possible to ignore the role of fathers in the parthenogenesis of psychiatric disorders, and asks 'what equally charming qualities these invisible fathers would manifest should we look for them' (Hors-fall, 1991: 233). Much of the first half of the twentieth century therefore involved a level of blaming mothers on two levels: for mental illness in their children more generally and for abuse of their children in particular, even for sexual abuse perpetrated by their husbands. Mothers effectively became the scapegoats *du jour* for psychiatry, psychology and social work during this period, with little recognition of male-perpetrated violence against women or children. The silence and mother-blame surrounding gendered violence and abuse was not to continue entirely unabated, though, because it was forcefully challenged by the second wave feminist movement in the 1960s and 1970s.

Gendered violence and second wave feminism

Feminists have been instrumental in bringing attention and recognition to sexual assault, child sexual abuse and domestic violence. As the women's movement gained momentum in the 1960s and 1970s, women's experiences of male-perpetrated violence and abuse began to emerge, often through consciousness-raising groups. Breckenridge (1999) points out that feminists at that time saw gender and power as central to these experiences, as had first wave feminists, and new services in Australia had an explicitly feminist orientation. Second wave feminism therefore made clear the links between male privilege and the violence and abuse experienced by women and children, with women narrating their own experiences of violence and, by so doing, demonstrating the connection between their life histories and wider gender inequalities (Reavey and Warner, 2003). Because gendered violence and abuse were seen to be common to many women's lives, the argument was made that they should not be seen as personal events for an unfortunate few but as a politico-social problem of patriarchy because they are 'endemic to all patriarchal societies that prioritise the needs of men in public as well as private life' (Reavey and Warner, 2003: 3). Thus, feminists were able to attack societies founded on male privilege that had been maintained by an imposed female silence (Reavey and Warner, 2003). In relation to child sexual abuse in particular, Haaken (2003) argues that, '[w]ithin feminism, the incest survivor's story was a project of stripping patriarchy of its fig leaf of benevolence to expose the violations of individual and collective father figures' (p. 81). While there was an awareness during this period that violence and abuse had a negative impact on women's psychological wellbeing, there was an understandable caution on the part of feminists about focusing on its mental health effects, particularly in relation to domestic violence, because of the risk of medicalisation and a shift away from justice concerns (Humphreys and Thiara, 2003). Dedicated feminist attention to the links between abuse and mental health problems came later in the 1980s as attention to child sexual abuse grew, while dedicated feminist attention to the mental health effects of domestic violence came even later.

Alongside the naming of male-perpetrated violence and abuse during second wave feminism, there was also growing attention from feminists to women's experiences of mental illness more generally during this period. Phillis Chesler's (2005) ground-breaking book *Women and Madness* was first published in 1972 and was one of the first in this area. While experiences of gendered violence and abuse were included in the stories from the women Chesler interviewed in the late 1960s and early 1970s, they were not the focus of her analysis. Chesler (2005) more broadly traced the historically higher prevalence of mental illness among women to patriarchy and misogyny or, in other words, to the complete devaluing of all things feminine. This, she argued, resulted in a 'slave psychology' for women based on servitude. Essentially, Chesler (2005) saw the social imposition of femininity on women *as* abuse, with mental illness an exaggerated form of, and capitulation to, presumed feminine frailty and dependence that often followed a woman's attempt to rebel against the constraints placed upon her. Chesler (2005) further argued that psychiatry colluded with patriarchy to force women into their feminine role, offering case examples where aggressive behaviour and other refusals of femininity resulted in women's incarceration in mental institutions with discharge dependent on the acceptance of femininity. Through its Freudian legacy, a focus on mothers remained in Chesler's work, though, and this also characterised much feminist scholarship on women and psychology during the 1970s and early 1980s. As such, there was little feminist attention to the role of gendered violence and abuse in women's mental health over this period.

The 1980s saw feminists in Australia and elsewhere increasingly focusing on the effects of child sexual abuse as a result of phone-ins and other opportunities for women to speak out (Breckenridge, 1999). Levett (2003) suggests that the concept of trauma was introduced by feminists as part of a critique of male power over women and adult power over girls. Therapeutic work with women who had histories of child sexual abuse became an increasing focus of practice for many social workers and other counsellors in feminist women's services, and awareness of sexual abuse as a form of male aggression against women and children remained pivotal to this. However, the 1990s saw a backlash against feminism (Faludi, 2006) and, along with it, a questioning of the veracity of reports of sexual abuse through the 'memory wars'. This was stimulated by the 'false memory syndrome' movement, largely driven by accused men, their partners and other apologists for sexual relations between adults and children. As Breckenridge (1999) points out, just as Freud had created disquiet and denial when he 'discovered' child sexual abuse, so had the feminist movement stirred this same pot through its revelations some 70 years later. Nonetheless, when feminists broke the silence on child sexual abuse in the 1980s, the 'child sexual abuse industry' was born (Armstrong, 1994) and mainstream psychology, psychiatry and medicine became increasingly involved in research into the connections between backgrounds of abuse and mental illness, and in the provision of treatment in this area. Most significantly, this industry has promulgated the idea of 'victim-illness' (Armstrong, 1994) and 'harm' (O'Dell, 2003), largely losing sight of feminist understandings of sexual assault as male aggression based on systems of male privilege and patriarchy (Armstrong, 1994). Thus, 'the metaphor of damage' introduced by feminists through the concept of trauma has shifted and 'in the context of professional and protection discourses of regulation and social control, the damaging effects of child sexual abuse become as factual as a broken bone' (Levett, 2003: 56). Moreover, Levett (2003) argues that this has become a justification for counterproductive interventions for children and families. Thus, professionals have reconstituted the political and social agenda of the women's movement into an individualistic, therapeutic one (Reavey and Warner, 2003) and abuse has become apolitical (Lamb, 1999). I now turn to examine how knowledge about the connections between abuse and mental illness has developed and proceeded alongside historical ebbs and flows of recognition and denial of gendered violence and abuse.

A global problem

The United Nations (UN) has defined violence against women as 'any act of gender-based violence that results in, or is likely to result in, physical, sexual or psychological harm or suffering to women, including threats of such acts, coercion or arbitrary deprivation of liberty, whether occurring in public or private life' (UN, 1993). Further to this, the World Health Organization (WHO) describes violence against women as 'a global public health problem of epidemic proportions, requiring urgent action' rather than a problem occurring only in some pockets of society' (WHO, 2013: 3). As noted earlier, the past four decades have seen a burgeoning of mainstream research into the links between gendered violence, abuse and mental health, particularly child sexual abuse. There has been a shift in psychiatric understandings of the origins of 'psychiatric illness' across the twentieth century, from fantasy to biology to actual events, so that adult mental health problems are now being linked to backgrounds of abuse (Nurnberg and Raskin, 1997). The enormous body of research that has grown up since the second wave feminist movement put gendered violence and abuse on the agenda overwhelmingly demonstrates that all forms of childhood abuse and domestic violence are associated with higher rates of mental health problems. Thus, individuals who have experienced abuse are over-represented in most categories of mental illness (for example, Chen *et al.*, 2010; Golding, 1999; Messman-Moore and Garrigus, 2007; O'Dougherty Wright *et al.*, 2009) and abuse appears to have a more negative impact on mental health for women (Downs and Miller, 1998; Itzin *et al.*, 2010).

I now turn to critically examine some of the evidence about the prevalence of gendered violence and abuse, and the connections to poor mental health and wellbeing. This body of research is positivist and quantitative, and the research into mental health treats 'mental illnesses' as real and distinctive entities, intelligible through psychiatric knowledge such as the *Diagnostic and Statistical Manual of Mental Disorders* (APA, 2013). As a feminist, I approach this literature with great caution and a critical perspective. More specifically, and as mentioned in the previous chapter, mainstream psycho-medical approaches have constructed a 'harm' story about abuse, child sexual abuse particularly (O'Dell,

2003), where permanent psychological damage is presumed to virtually always occur. This is a powerful story with myriad implications for women and children as its main subjects. I have no wish to participate in cementing this story further or extending it to other forms of abuse. However, I nonetheless argue that it is important to outline some of the central claims of mainstream research in this area as part of the strategic feminist project of acknowledging the depth and breadth of emotional distress caused to many (not all) women and children by gendered violence and abuse, but also by the ways it is understood and theorised. Thus, while I do not share any of the pathologising assumptions of the psycho-medical discourses and practices on which this knowledge is based, neither do I want to dismiss out of hand what some of the more rigorous research might allude to about the levels of women's (and children's) distress.

Child sexual abuse

As for all gendered violence and abuse, it is difficult to accurately assess the extent of child sexual abuse because most cases never come to the attention of authorities as a result of silencing, stigma and continuing socio-cultural taboos. We are therefore left with estimations of prevalence that are mainly based on cross-sectional self-report research with all of the potential methodological problems and limitations these types of studies involve. Estimations of the extent of child sexual abuse vary widely depending on the way abuse is defined and the data collection methods used. Thus, some studies use looser definitions, such as any unwanted sexual experience before 18 years of age, while others require touching or sexual intercourse. Some also impose age restrictions such as more than a five-year difference between the abused and the abuser. Briere and Runtz (1988) reported a rate of approximately 15 per cent among women in the United States using a definition of abuse as sexual contact involving touching between a girl 15 years or under and a perpetrator at least five years older. In a widely reported meta-analysis from the United States, Bolen and Scannapieco (1999) found prevalence rates from 23–40 per cent for females and 3–13 per cent for males. Stoltenborgh *et al.* (2011) conducted a meta-analysis of prevalence figures for child sexual abuse studies from around the world, published between 1980 and 2008, and found prevalence rates of 18 per cent for girls and 4 per cent for boys, with most studies using a five-year age difference between abused and abuser as their definition. These authors concluded that child sexual abuse is a global problem of considerable proportions. The key point to take away from these diverse prevalence rates is that whichever measure is used, girls are two to three times more likely to be sexually abused than boys (May-Chahal, 2006). Moreover, the perpetrators are far and away more likely to be male (Dhaliwal *et al.*, 1996; Romano and De Luca, 2001), irrespective of the sex of the child, with men comprising approximately 95 per cent of sexual offenders in the UK (British Department of Health (DH), cited in Warner, 2009).

The body of research connecting child sexual abuse with adult mental health problems is particularly vast. I provide only a brief overview of some of the key findings here, with most of the cited studies cross-sectional, retrospective and conducted in either Australia, the United Kingdom or the United States. A number of studies have identified associations between child sexual abuse and post-traumatic stress disorder (PTSD) (Briggs and Joyce, 1997; Canton-Cortes and Canton, 2010; Shakespeare-Finch and De Dassel, 2009); anxiety disorders (Briere and Runtz, 1988; Chaffin *et al.*, 2005; Mennen and Meadow, 1995; Saunders *et al.*, 1992; Stein *et al.*, 1996); depression (Briere and Runtz, 1988; Mennen and Meadow, 1995; Spataro *et al.*, 2004); panic disorder (Leskin and Sheikh, 2002); agoraphobia (Saunders *et al.*, 1992); eating disorders (Carter *et al.*, 2006; Chen *et al.*, 2010); 'personality disorders'[1] (Spataro *et al.*, 2004); suicidal behaviour (Curtis, 2006); and poorer mental health in general (Fleming *et al.*, 1999; Najman *et al.*, 2007). In some estimates, childhood sexual abuse has been estimated to increase an individual's risk of anxiety by as much as five times and depression by as much as four times (Briere and Elliot, 1994). Trickett *et al.* (2011) conducted a 23-year longitudinal study in the United States, a particularly robust quantitative method, to examine the impact of intra-familial child sexual abuse on women, linking abuse to PTSD, depression, so-called 'cognitive deficits', dissociative symptoms, 'maladaptive sexual development', self-harm, drug and alcohol abuse, physical health problems and a host of social problems such as 'teen motherhood'. However, Najman *et al.* (2007) emphasise that while their research found that child sexual abuse has negative effects on mental and physical health for many individuals, it also found that some individuals do not experience problems.

Many of the above studies find that women's mental health problems are more severe when the abuser is older (Briere and Runtz, 1988); when there are multiple abusers (Briere and Runtz, 1988); when abusers are relatives (Briere and Runtz, 1988; Hulme and Agrawal, 2004), especially father figures (Mennen and Meadow, 1995); if abuse is of long duration or is repeated (Briere and Runtz, 1988, Briggs and Joyce, 1997); when abuse is more severe (Chaffin *et al.*, 2005); if force is used (Hulme and Agrawal, 2004); and if penetration occurs (Briere and Runtz, 1988; Briggs and Joyce, 1997; Mennen and Meadow, 1995). Moreover, certain types of sexual abuse have been found to be associated with the most serious mental health problems, particularly ongoing intra-familial abuse, and these are more likely to be experienced by girls (May-Chahal, 2006). It has been argued that girls and women are therefore more likely to experience high levels of betrayal because of the nature of the abuse they experience, thereby influencing the nature of their distress (Freyd, 1997). As noted earlier, there is evidence that child sexual abuse has more deleterious mental health consequences for girls and women (Itzin *et al.*, 2010), although other influential socio-cultural discourses and practices frame these experiences and are examined further later in terms of their implications for women's mental health and wellbeing.

Childhood emotional abuse

As noted earlier, recognition of childhood emotional abuse has been much more recent, in part related to difficulties in defining it, but it is attracting increasing attention there's growing recognition of child abuse more generally. Unfortunately, childhood emotional abuse is in some ways distinguished by its very ordinariness and banality. As is pointed out by Boulton and Hindle (2000), the qualitative aspects of emotional abuse can be found in most parenting and caregiving between adults and children. However, for these to be considered abuse, they must be pervasive, persistent and inflexible (Boulton and Hindle, 2000). In spite of difficulties in defining childhood emotional abuse, a widely accepted definition suggests that it involves 'a verbal assault on a child's sense of worth and wellbeing, or any humiliating, demeaning or threatening behaviour directed toward a child by an older person' (Bernstein and Fink, 1998: 2).

Emerging quantitative evidence reveals that childhood emotional abuse is the most common form of child abuse (Australian Institute of Health and Welfare (AIHW), 2014; Stoltenborgh, 2012). One-third of US college students report a history of some form of child abuse with one-third reporting childhood emotional abuse (Braver *et al.*, 1992). O'Dougherty Wright *et al.* (2009) report rates of 5.6 to 34.8 per cent from their review of studies, depending on the type of definitions and methods used. More specifically, of the 53,666 cases of substantiated child abuse in Australia between 2012 and 2013, 38 per cent involved childhood emotional abuse (AIHW, 2014). Claussen and Crittenden (1991) also suggest that emotional abuse may underlie other forms of abuse as a 'core issue' (Claussen and Crittenden, 1991), and this will be elaborated further later. Of the limited research that is available, it appears that both fathers and mothers perpetrate childhood emotional abuse, with fathers somewhat more likely to be perpetrators (Sedlak *et al.*, 2010). There is also some evidence that experiences of childhood emotional abuse are more commonly reported by women and girls, with rates ranging from 8 to 14.3 per cent for girls and 4 to 9.6 per cent for boys (Cawson *et al.*, 2000; Scher *et al.*, 2004), and girls commonly report higher rates particularly within the family (Cawson *et al.*, 2000). Scher *et al.* (2004) report that in a community sample, rather than a clinical one, childhood emotional abuse was approximately 14 per cent for women and 9.6 per cent for men. Downs and Miller (1998) found that fathers' verbal aggression and physical violence, and its severity, predicted psychiatric symptomology in daughters but not in sons, whereas mothers' abuse did not predict problems in either daughters or sons. However, while gender differences in self-reported prevalence have been noted, few suggestions have been offered for why girls might report more emotional abuse or why the effects on mental health seem to be more severe. Lastly, childhood emotional abuse often occurs in the context of other child abuse (O'Dougherty Wright *et al.*, 2009) and with parental alcoholism and other family problems (Dong *et al.*, 2004). Mullen *et al.* (1996) show that all forms of abuse are more common in conflicted families who experience social disadvantage, although such families are also subject to greater surveillance by child protection agencies (May-Chahal, 2006). However, while childhood emotional abuse may be highly prevalent, it is also the most hidden and underreported form of abuse.

Childhood emotional abuse is increasingly linked by researchers to poor mental health (O'Dougherty Wright *et al.*, 2009). Mental health conditions that have been specifically linked to childhood emotional abuse are wide-ranging and include increased anxiety and depression (Mullen *et al.*, 1996; Spertus *et al.*, 2003); PTSD (Spertus *et al.*, 2003), personality disorders (Johnson *et al.*, 1999); eating disorders (Kennedy *et al.*, 2007; Kent *et al.*, 1999; Fischer *et al.*, 2010); and schizophrenia (Cheavens *et al.*, 2005). Moreover, the mental health effects of childhood emotional abuse have been shown to often persist into old age (Sachs-Ericsson *et al.*, 2010). Childhood emotional abuse is also more strongly and consistently linked to poor mental health than other forms of abuse (Schneider *et al.*, 2007; O'Dougherty Wright *et al.*, 2009). However, it is also thought to be particularly harmful when it occurs alongside other forms of abuse (O'Dougherty Wright *et al.*, 2009; Briere and Runtz, 1988), particularly sexual abuse (Messman-Moore and Garrigus, 2007), which can be thought of as inherently emotionally abusive in and of itself. Child physical abuse has also been associated with mental health problems such as anxiety (Stein *et al.*, 1996), however the links with poor mental health are not as clear-cut as for other forms of abuse particularly when sexual and emotional abuse are not involved. Thus, multiple types of abuse have been shown to be associated with the more serious mental health problems (Messman-Moore and Garrigus, 2007). However, like sexual abuse, it is also important to point out that not all individuals who experience childhood emotional abuse go on to experience mental health problems, with protective factors in the child's environment also identified as important (Glaser, 2011).

Domestic violence

In 2013, the WHO undertook the first global systematic review of prevalence data on violence against women, specifically domestic violence and sexual violence (WHO, 2013). The WHO estimates that, worldwide, 'almost one third of women who have been in a relationship have experienced physical and/or sexual violence by their intimate partner', with higher rates of 38 per cent in some regions (WHO, 2013: 2). This is an extremely large proportion of women across the world, particularly in view of the fact that some common forms of abuse experienced by women and girls are not included in this figure, such as emotional abuse in domestic violence and child sexual abuse. Moreover, it is estimated that 38 per cent of all murders of women worldwide are perpetrated by male partners (WHO, 2013). The 2012 Personal Safety Survey conducted in Australia has estimated that almost 41 per cent of women had experienced some form of physical violence since 15 years of age, mostly from someone known to them, such as an intimate partner (ABS, 2012). It has been estimated that for 62 per cent of women, the most recent incident of physical violence was experienced at the hands of a male in their home, drawing attention to the fact that domestic violence against women is also perpetrated by other male family members in addition to partners (ABS, 2012). In a 12-month period, 10 per cent of women in Australia are affected by domestic violence, increasing to 20 per cent when measured across the life course (ABS, 2006). In 2009, the National Council to

Reduce Violence Against Women and their Children and KPMG Management Consulting (2009) estimated that violence against women and children cost the Australian economy $13.6 billion per year. Domestic violence occurs across all age groups, cultures and socio-economic groups in Australia, with Indigenous Australian women most vulnerable (Davis and Taylor, 2002). While much prevalence research on domestic violence focuses on physical and sexual violence, it is widely accepted that domestic violence includes physical, psychological/emotional, sexual, financial and social abuse, the use of children and pets, and threats and intimidation (DeKeseredy, 2011), with each type distinguished by the effort to control women (Stark, 2007; WHO, 2013). While there have been claims over the last two decades that domestic violence is 'gender symmetrical', meaning that just as many men are victims as women, this is not borne out by any of the research that distinguishes the severity of violence, fear in victims and the impact of violence (Dobash *et al.*, 1992; Allen Walby and Allen, 2004, both cited in Walby *et al.*, 2014), with the great majority of severe and ongoing domestic violence perpetrated by men against women (Itzin *et al.*, 2012). Tactics of coercive control particularly distinguish domestic violence perpetrated by men against their female partners (see Stark, 2007).

Attention to the mental health consequences of domestic violence has been more recent. There is now a large body of research specifically linking domestic violence with poor mental health for women. In the systematic review of global prevalence data conducted by the WHO and referred to earlier, it is estimated that women who experience domestic violence are twice as likely to experience depression (WHO, 2013). A meta-analysis conducted by Golding (1999) shows very high rates of PTSD, depression, suicidality, alcohol abuse and drug abuse across the studies considered. Stark and Flitcraft (1996) argue that a sense of entrapment can often lead women to attempt suicide. Golding (1999) has gone so far as to argue that a causal relationship exists between domestic violence and poor mental health for women based on the compelling evidence from his meta-analysis of self-harm, depression and PTSD. Other studies have also linked domestic violence to anxiety (for example, McCauley *et al.*, 1995). Some studies have also shown that when compared to women with no histories of domestic violence, women who report both past and current violence are almost six times more likely to report psychological distress (Romito *et al.*, 2005). Others studies have shown that, as for childhood abuse, experiencing multiple forms of abuse (for example, physical, psychological/emotional and sexual abuse) increases the severity of mental health problems (Bonomi *et al.*, 2009). Lastly, Walby (2004) asserts that the heavier burden of poor mental health carried by women is at least in part traceable to domestic violence.

The rise in trauma models

The WHO suggests that the increased risks of mental health problems associated with violence against women is related to 'traumatic stress' (WHO, 2013). Trauma and PTSD are now such widespread terms that some commentators suggest we are in 'the age of trauma' (Miller and Tougaw, 2002: 1, cited in Tseris, 2013: 155), and this is particularly the case in research and practice focused on gendered violence and abuse. Since the early 1990s, trauma models have been increasingly applied to understandings of the effects of child sexual abuse, while their application to the impact of child emotional abuse and domestic violence have been more recent (Humphreys and Thiara, 2003; Spertus *et al.*, 2003). In the most recent version of the *Diagnostic and Statistical Manual of Mental Disorders* (DSM) (APA, 2013), PTSD has been reclassified as trauma rather than as an anxiety disorder (APA, 2013). It is described as triggered by being exposed to actual or threatened death, sexual assault or serious injury, and as characterised by re-experiencing the trauma, avoidance, negative cognitions and mood, and arousal (APA, 2013). Unlike other psychiatric diagnoses, PTSD potentially acknowledges the role of violence and abuse in individual distress and therefore places the causes outside the individual and in their situation. However, as noted earlier in relation to child sexual abuse in particular, there is now a 'harm story' of abuse in the psycho-medical literature, which constructs a 'highly singu-larised "story" of psychological harm in which one story speaks for all women's experiences' (O'Dell, 2003: 131). Arguably, this story of harm has been extended to other forms of child abuse and more recently to domestic violence, too. In the next section, I consider both the benefits and problems of the trauma models, however, I also critically engage with specific trauma models as they have been applied to the specific mental health problems considered in subsequent chapters.

Contemporary feminist approaches

Since the second wave women's movement put gendered violence and abuse squarely on the social agenda, feminist researchers have created a formidable repository of scholarly work that has challenged many of the assumptions and blind-spots of mainstream research in this area. This work is wide-ranging and includes feminist psychological approaches to trauma, post-structural feminist research into the effects of child sexual abuse and more materialist and realist structural feminist approaches to women's mental health in the context of domestic violence.

Feminist approaches to trauma

As noted earlier, feminists first appropriated and used the concept of trauma as part of a critique of male power over women and adult power over girls. Seminal work developing a feminist trauma approach to understanding and working with women who have experienced gendered violence and abuse was undertaken in the United States by the well-known feminist psychiatrist, Judith Herman. In her first book, *Father-Daughter Incest*, first published in 1981, Herman (2000) criti-cally examines from a feminist perspective the sexual abuse of girls by fathers and other male relatives, and the harm it causes. Herman (2000) links incest to 'the ideology of male dominance' (p. 22) and in a move highly progressive and ground-breaking for its time, she sets out to show in no uncertain terms the cata-logue of harms that commonly flow from intra-familial child sexual abuse based on her research with 40 women from her clinical practice. Herman (2000) unequivocally centres the question of power in her theorisation of incest, point-ing out that children cannot refuse a sexual advance from an adult, particularly from a parent, and that such a 'relationship' always involves elements of coer-cion, with many men able to exploit the power imbalance without resorting to outright force. She shows that many women report feeling stigmatised and shameful as if 'the incest secret formed the core of their identity' (Herman, 2000: 97). It is in her second book, *Trauma and Recovery*, that Herman (1997) embraces the psychological construct of 'trauma', expanding on it and re-working it to feminist ends. She provides a highly refined and nuanced under-standing of the specific nature of psychological trauma caused by violence and abuse against women and children, taking a broader approach by including all types of abuse, not just child sexual abuse. Herman (1997) draws a compelling analogy between the trauma caused by war, torture and imprisonment and that caused by gendered violence and abuse. She points out that it was the study of combat neurosis after the world wars that developed a body of knowledge about traumatic disorders. This was because there was little awareness of the routine nature of violence and abuse in women's day-to-day lives and, as shown earlier, retreat and denial when this reality was glimpsed by psychiatrists such as Freud (Herman, 1997). Herman (1997) shows how many of the symptoms experienced by women and children following rape, sexual abuse and male-perpetrated phys-ical violence mirror those described by combat veterans, and she goes on to argue that '[t]here is war between the sexes. Rape victims, battered women, and sexually abused children are its casualties. Hysteria is the combat neurosis of the sex war' (Herman, 1997: 32). Herman (1997) suggests that the traumas of the public realm of war and those of the private domestic world are the same, that is, that 'the hysteria of women and the combat neurosis of men are one' (p. 32). Herman (1997) makes a case for a new category of post-traumatic stress disorder – complex post-traumatic stress disorder (c-PTSD) – that acknowledges the spe-cific psychological trauma wrought by gendered violence and abuse. While the proposed condition of c-PTSD has not been accepted by the American Psycho-logical Association and it therefore remains outside the current *Diagnostic and Statistical Manual of Mental Disorders*, many feminist clinicians and researchers nonetheless draw on and apply the concept in their work with abused women.

Herman's work draws on a radical feminist understanding where gendered violence and abuse reflect men's desire to terrorise and oppress women into sub-mission, including sexual submission, with an understanding of patriarchy as the frame for violence against women. However, alongside this, she relies on main-stream psychological theories of abnormal development and psychopathology to explain how abuse severs assumed 'normal developmental pathways' for women. Thus, while Herman brings a feminist eye to women's experiences of gendered violence and abuse and its impact on their lives, and there is great empathy and understanding in her writing, as in mainstream trauma theory, women are nonetheless pathologised as psychologically damaged although not inevitably nor irrevocably so.

The concepts of trauma and the diagnostic category of PTSD have been increasingly adopted by feminist practitioners and researchers to understand and work with the emotional consequences of all types of gendered violence and abuse. In her critique of contemporary feminist adoptions of trauma theory, Tseris (2013) argues that approaches are often deterministic about the effects of abuse and violence on women's lives, with neurobiological theories increasingly used that devalue social change and activism. Gavey (2003) argues that some psychological explanations of trauma, such as John Briere's (2002) 'self-trauma model', is embraced by many feminist practitioners because it is sympathetic, nuanced and not far off feminist social constructionist approaches to understanding women's strategies for coping with sexual abuse as 'survival strategies'. However, there is a risk that trauma models, especially those emphasising neurobiology, may bolster biological knowledge and devalue women's narratives of their experiences, centring 'the brain' rather than 'the self': indeed, neurobiological research is already being used to deeply pathologise supposed 'deficits' in abused children (Tseris, 2013). Moreover, as many commentators have pointed out, gendered violence and abuse are distinctive for their more chronic nature, and for the fact that the abusers are known to, and usually related to, the abused woman (for example, Briere and Lanktree, 2012): as such, profound feelings of betrayal can be important (see Freyd, 1997) as well as the specific gender discourses and the wider power relations that frame gendered violence and abuse. Nonetheless, Tseris (2013) points out that some feminists have used the diagnosis of PTSD or c-PTSD as a compromise between deficit psychiatric approaches and feminist understandings of gender inequality and mental health. In the research I present later in this book, I show that many women themselves also embrace the diagnosis of PTSD as opposed to other psychiatric approaches to labelling their distress. However, there are tensions related to this, including the tendency to obscure social justice issues and the actions of perpetrators, which I address further in Chapter 8.

Feminist approaches to child sexual abuse and mental health

Post-structural feminist research and scholarship about child sexual abuse is probably the largest body of work on gendered violence, abuse and mental health. Most of this work comes from feminist critical psychologists Reavey and Warner (2003), O'Dell (2003), Warner and Wilkins (2003) and Warner (2009). Reavey and Warner (2003) have brought together feminist scholars and practitioners to explore new feminist stories of child sexual abuse as opposed to the standard stories of pathology and victimhood. The different contributions have in common the effort to make visible discourses about sex, gender and childhood that commonly underpin explanations of child sexual abuse and its effects. The important point is made by Reavey (2003) and by Warner and Wilkins (2003) that many of the symptoms of child sexual abuse identified in women are also associated with 'femininity' more generally, that is, irrationality, powerlessness and unreasonableness. However, the assumptions about gender that underlie the identification of these supposed traits are never flagged and remain hidden in the mainstream literature (Reavey, 2003).

Two other chapters, one by O'Dell (2003) and the other by Warner and Wilkins (2003), specifically report on the authors' research into child sexual abuse and mental health. O'Dell (2003) undertook interviews with professionals who worked with children or adults with histories of child sexual abuse, and women who identified as 'survivors' of child sexual abuse. O'Dell (2003) shows how a discourse of development enables a positioning of women and children as products of their abusive pasts, with abuse seen as disrupting this developmental pathway so that the abused child becomes 'other' to the non-abused 'normal' child, and women become lifelong victims (O'Dell, 2003). O'Dell (2003) identifies powerful discourses of developmentalism in professionals' talk, including the idea that later life events 'trigger' the effects of abuse, with women positioned as harmed for the rest of their lives. O'Dell (2003) shows that the harm story is therefore totalising, but it is also revealed to be partial, gendered, heterosexualised and raced (class is not mentioned), with all of these issues either oversimplified or rendered invisible.

Warner and Wilkins (2003) undertook research in a British secure hospital with both patients and professional staff to examine intersections between explanations of women patients, the diagnosis of borderline personality disorder and histories of child sexual abuse. They demonstrate how the act of diagnosis is central to regulating patients and professionals, determining who is 'abnormal' and who can speak of it legitimately, and perhaps revealing more about 'ideologies and social hierarchical social structures than about the "disorders" of which they ostensibly speak' (Warner and Wilkins, 2003: 172). They point out the way that 'symptoms' of borderline personality disorder, such as emotional lability, rage, self-destructiveness, depression and feelings of emptiness, are also commonly associated with 'normative femininity' (Warner and Wilkins, 2003: 172). They argue that it is therefore unsurprising that women are much more likely to meet the criteria than men. Many women who are given this diagnosis also have histories of child sexual abuse, and they go on to point out that both child sexual abuse and borderline personality disorder are gender-saturated narratives (Warner and Wilkins, 2003). Thus, borderline personality disorder 'can be understood as the social embodiment of child sexual abuse, as well as (already pathologised) femininity' (Warner and Wilkins, 2003: 172). As in O'Dell's (2003) research, child sexual abuse is explained by professionals as causing disruption to the personality structure in the form of 'fragmentation'. Warner and Wilkins (2003) argue that understanding borderline symptoms and child sexual abuse could socially locate women's actions and normalise their behaviour. However, this has not usually occurred in the case of borderline personality disorder because the process of diagnosis works to obscure the social dimensions of traumatisation, primarily because this condition is framed around emotions and not abuse. I suggest that the failure to produce a social account of traumatisation is not necessarily because the process of diagnosis centres emotion per se, but because psychiatry has a pathologised and individualised understanding of emotion (and of 'diagnosis' for that matter) as symptomatic only of illness in the individual, particularly in women. I propose a more sociological understanding of emotion for the purposes of my own research in the following chapter.

Warner (2009) presents more detailed findings of her study into the ways language impacts on shaping the experiences of sexually abused women in secure mental health care in the UK in her later sole-authored book. Warner shows how this focus on personality enables workers to avoid the problems of childhood sexual abuse and self-harm. Warner (2009) also shows how the 'normal' woman is understood to be caring of others, sensible, responsible, not aggressive, hopeful and as having 'insight'. Thus, Warner (2009) shows the workings of gender discourses in workers' and women's accounts of mental illness and child sexual abuse, often with highly contradictory assumptions. She argues that the whole debate must be shifted to asking questions about the worlds women live in rather than making assumptions about 'what's gone wrong in their heads' (Warner, 2009: 139), and she particularly emphasises the role of betrayal in women's experiences. Post-structural feminist research into child sexual abuse and mental health has therefore elaborated the ways that gender discourses structure both the explanations of abuse and the theories used to explain women's mental health problems.

Childhood emotional abuse: building towards a gender perspective

As noted in the introductory chapter, childhood emotional abuse has not yet received any attention from feminist researchers. As demonstrated above, child sexual abuse and domestic violence are experienced by many more women and girls than men and boys, with men far more likely to be the perpetrators. As such, these problems can be relatively unproblematically understood as gendered, although their gendered dimensions are far more complex than this. Childhood emotional abuse is not so clearly gendered in the sense of the gender of perpetrators because both men *and* women are commonly perpetrators. So how can it be argued, then, that childhood emotional abuse is gendered in this most usual sense of the word? While there has been no feminist consideration of childhood emotional abuse, there has been some feminist attention to child physical abuse, which is also reported relatively evenly between the genders both for victimisation and perpetration (May-Chahal, 2006), and some of the insights may have relevance to child emotional abuse, too. While women are said to perpetrate child physical abuse in relatively equal numbers to men, the fact that they spend far more time with their children is often taken into account as a mitigating factor (Featherstone, 1997; Straus *et al.*, 1998, cited in May-Chahal, 2006), and this is also likely to be relevant to some child emotional abuse. However, May-Chahal (2006) argues that this is only a partial explanation of the gender dimensions of this type of child abuse. She suggests that the problem with much mainstream research into child abuse is that it fails to address the meanings of both 'abuse' and 'gender', treating them only as uni-dimensional variables of measurement rather than 'acknowledging gendered social relations and violence in their situated contexts' (May-Chahal, 2006: 53). May-Chahal (2006) points to an early feminist study by Graham (1980), which showed that anger, frustration and aggression were the norm among mothers caring for infant children, with the author concluding that the more pressing question is why more women do not assault their children than why a small proportion do (Graham, 1980, cited in May-Chahal, 2006). May-Chahal (2006) argues that the expectation that it is mothers who have the duty of care to children, and mothers who are the focus of child protection agencies, is also relevant to understanding the gender dimensions of child physical abuse. She cites Australian research by Thorpe and Jackson (1997), where the researchers delved behind child abuse statistics to discover why so many women were identified as physically violent to their children when women are under-represented in other forms of violence. They found that many cases were not substantiated by child protection agencies and that the large numbers of women reported were more reflective of the surveillance of child-rearing practices and motherhood than with risks to children (Thorpe and Jackson, 1997, cited in May-Chahal, 2006). Instead, the researchers show that a substantial proportion of the cases involved excessive use of corporal punishment to discipline children in order to socialise them (Thorpe and Jackson, 1997, cited in May-Chahal, 2006). It is quite likely that such 'discipline' can also involve emotional abuse in the form of verbal abuse, too. According to May-Chahal (2006), in some European jurisdictions, harsh treatment such as this has been reframed as 'excessive care relations' rather than 'abuse', and this has been seen as descriptive of the child-rearing practices of some mothers as well as fathers, with class and culture also relevant. What May-Chahal (2006) shows is that child physical abuse is framed by gender in complex ways, where mothers' responsibilities are over-emphasised while fathers are often divested of responsibility, and that this occurs in the context of gendered social relations, as well as those of class and race.

These insights into child physical abuse are arguably relevant to those aspects of childhood emotional abuse that might be concerned with 'discipline', but it is perhaps naive to seek to explain away all non-sexual child abuse as 'socialisation'. Other 'non-disciplinary' practices such as scapegoating are also part of child emotional abuse (Moran *et al.*, 2002). Whatever way childhood emotional abuse might be understood, it has nonetheless been unequivocally linked with particularly negative mental health outcomes. Moreover, childhood emotional abuse seems to be reported more often by girls and women, although not to the same levels of gender asymmetry as for sexual abuse and domestic violence; it appears to have more serious consequences when it is perpetrated by fathers against daughters; and it often occurs alongside sexual abuse. As feminists, then, there is arguably a moral imperative to further investigate the possible gendered dimensions of childhood emotional abuse. What is particularly striking about the existing mainstream research into childhood emotional abuse is not only that it largely ignores gender, as does most of the research into gendered violence and abuse, but that it never attends to *what* is actually said and done, by *who* or *where*, that is, to the content, power relations and contexts of abuse. All of the quantitative research in this area uses pre-determined scales that group abusive behaviours together. For example, Kennedy *et al.* (2007) report a direct unmediated relationship between childhood emotional abuse and eating pathology using a scale that asks if respondents experienced insulting, threatening and behaviour blaming, but inquire no further into the nature of the abuse. Cheavens *et al.* (2005) specify criticising, minimising, trivialising, punishing, erratic reinforcing of thoughts and feelings, and over-simplifying the ease of problem-solving as constitutive of emotional abuse, but the content or context of abuse is never alluded to. The research presented in Chapter 4 of this book therefore represents the first attempt to examine the gendered dimensions of childhood emotional abuse by specifically examining the gendered meanings and contexts of this type of abuse, and how it is framed by gendered discourses and gender power relations. The research shows that child emotional abuse involves profoundly gendered dimensions that have implications for how women and men overcome its emotional impact in their lives.

Materialist feminism, gendered violence and mental health

As noted earlier, dedicated feminist attention to women's mental health in the context of domestic violence is quite recent. This research largely emanates from feminist social work and public health and is primarily framed by a materialist feminist approach that centres women's lived experiences and situates them in gender power inequalities. As such, this research often assumes a relatively unproblematic relationship between what women say and their actual lived experiences. As part of a mixed methods study of PTSD after intimate partner violence, Scheffer Lindgren and Renck (2008) interviewed 14 women in Sweden about their experiences. They found that themes of fear/uncertainty and shame/ guilt were common, with participants describing psychological and sexual abuse as causing the deepest and longer term problems. In particular, the authors emphasise that prior to violence, many of the women regarded themselves as strong people, with the violence therefore experienced as particularly shocking. The study also showed that women with histories of trauma prior to domestic violence, including sexual abuse, found it more difficult to leave domestic violence. In Australia, Laing and Toivonen (2010) undertook a qualitative interview study with women about the impact of domestic violence on their mental health. Many women indicated that the controlling nature of the relationships they were in, and the ongoing knocks to their self-esteem, led to depression, panic attacks, PTSD, insomnia and suicidal actions. The mental health problems of panic and anxiety are directly linked in this research to women's experiences of a felt sense of relative powerlessness and inequality in relation to their partners (Laing and Toivonen, 2010). In the UK, Humphreys and Thiara (2003) surveyed and interviewed women, and showed that they articulated a direct, causal relationship between domestic violence and their mental health problems. Humphreys and

Thiara (2003) offer examples where women described losing their confidence and self-worth by being worn down by abuse and being made to believe they were inferior to their partners. They show the extreme control exerted on women by their violent partners, borrowing Johnson and Ferraro's (2000) concept of 'intimate terrorism' and suggesting that the men have attempted to 'eradicate the women's sense of self and create instead a "puppet woman" subject to their authority' (Humphreys and Thiara, 2003: 215). They argue that male control such as this is the contextual frame for the suicide attempts described by some of the women in their study. Further to this, the authors argue that the medical model can 'sever the link between abuse and emotional distress' so that 'the focus shifts from the man and his responsibility for what are often criminal acts of violence and abuse to the woman and her mental health problems' (Humphreys and Thiara, 2003: 219). Humphreys and Thiara (2003) conclude that, nonetheless, the diagnostic category of PTSD can be preferable to women than other diagnoses because it at least acknowledges the link between abuse and distress. I return to this complex question later.

In an effort to approach gendered violence and abuse in an interconnected way, Itzin *et al.* (2010) undertook feminist research in the UK into domestic violence, sexual violence and abuse, and their connections with health and mental health for women. This research was framed by a public health approach and the view that physical, emotional and sexual abuse, childhood neglect and domestic violence cause mental and physical ill-health in children, adolescents and adults, mainly women. Itzin *et al.* (2010) use Heise's (1998) multidimensional 'ecological framework' where violence and abuse are viewed as resulting from a complex interaction of factors operating at four levels: individual, including 'personality factors'; immediate relationships; community, including social and peer networks, workplaces and neighbourhoods; and society, meaning the macro-system and cultural values, beliefs and practices (Itzin *et al.*, 2010). They describe the findings of a consultation project undertaken as part of the Victims of Violence and Abuse Prevention Programme (VVAPP) where they consulted with large numbers of practitioners and community members about the principles, values and core beliefs of best-practice in this area. They also undertook a systematic review of the literature on the epidemiology, impact, therapeutic intervention, protection and prevention strategies. Like other structural and more realist feminist work into domestic violence and mental health, Itzin *et al.* (2010) give voice to women's experiences and emphasise the serious consequences of violence for women. This type of feminist research has also, importantly, shown how unequal power and control are integral to the negative mental health impact of gendered violence and abuse, challenging pathologising medical assumptions by raising social factors above individual ones.

A rich repository of feminist research into gendered violence, abuse and mental health clearly exists, bringing diverse perspectives and insights that challenge some of the pathologising assumptions of psycho-medical approaches. The most powerful challenge to psycho-medical discourses about abused women comes from post-structural feminist research into the effects of child sexual abuse, while other feminist research into domestic violence and mental health has given voice to women's lived experiences and draws attention to unequal gender power relations in the emergence of women's emotional distress in contexts of violence. As yet, there has been no feminist research into childhood emotional abuse at all, necessitating an extension of feminist attention to this area. In the following chapters, I aim to build on feminist research into gendered violence, abuse and mental health by considering together the discursive and material dimensions of women's experiences, situating this in the wider context of gender inequalities that continue to frame women's day-to-day lives. In the next chapter, I explain how I charted a course between discursive and materialist feminist traditions by attending both to the symbolic dimensions of women's experiences and to their material lived experiences of gendered violence, abuse and mental health in contexts of unequal gender power relations.

Note

1 I use parentheses for some of the more pejorative, pathologising terms used in this literature such as 'personality disorders', 'maladaptive sexual development', 'cognitive deficits' and 'teen motherhood'.

References

American Psychiatric Association (APA) (2013) *Diagnostic and Statistical Manual of Mental Disorders – DSM-5*. Arlington: APA.

Armstrong, L. (1994) *Rocking the Cradle of Sexual Politics: What Happened When Women Said Incest?* London: The Women's Press.

Australian Bureau of Statistics (ABS) (2006) *Personal Safety Survey* (reissue) Cat. No. 4906.0. Canberra.

Australian Bureau of Statistics (ABS) (2012) *Personal Safety*, Australia, 2012, 4906.0. Canberra.

Australian Institute of Health and Welfare (AIHW) (2014) *Child Protection Australia 2012–2013*. Canberra: Australian Government. Available at: www.aihw.gov.au/publication-detail/?id=60129547965, accessed 22 April 2015.

Bell, S. (2011) Through a Foucauldian lens: a geneology of child abuse, *Journal of Family Violence*, 26, pp. 101–108.

Bernstein, D.P. and Fink, L. (1998) *Childhood Trauma Questionnaire: A Retrospective Self-Report*. San Antonio: The Psychological Corporation.

Bolen, R.M. and Scannapieco, M. (1999) Prevalence of child sexual abuse: a corrective meta-analysis, *Social Service Review*, 73, pp. 281–313.

Bonomi, A.E., Anderson, M.L., Reid, R.J., Rivara, F.P., Carrell, D. and Thompson, R.S. (2009) Medical and psychosocial diagnoses in women with a history of intimate partner violence, *Archives of Internal Medicine*, 169(18), pp. 1692–1697.

Boulton, S. and Hindle, D. (2000) Emotional abuse: the work of a multidisciplinary consultation group in a child psychiatric service, *Clinical Child Psychology and Psychiatry*, 5(3), pp. 439–452.

Braver, M., Bumberry, J., Green, K. and Rawson, R. (1992) Childhood abuse and current psychological functioning in a university counseling center population, *Journal of Counseling Psychology*, 39(2), pp. 252–257.

Breckenridge, J. (1999) Subjugation and silences: the role of the professions in silencing victims of sexual and domestic violence. In J. Breckenridge and L. Laing (eds), *Challenging Silence: Innovative Responses to Sexual and Domestic Violence*. Sydney: Allen & Unwin, pp. 6–30.

Briere, J. (2002) Treating adult survivors of severe childhood abuse and neglect: further development of an integrative model. In J.E.B. Myers, L. Berliner, J. Briere, C.T. Hendrix, C. Jenny and T.A. Reid (eds), *The APSAC Handbook on Child Maltreatment*, second edition. Thousand Oaks: Sage Publications, pp. 175–203.

Briere, J. and Elliot, D.M. (1994) Immediate and long-term impacts of child sexual abuse, *The Future of Children: Sexual Abuse of Children*, 4(2), pp. 54–69.

Briere, J.N. and Lanktree, C.B. (2012) *Treating Complex Trauma in Adolescents and Young Adults*. Thousand Oaks: Sage.

Briere, J. and Runtz, M. (1988) Symptomatology associated with childhood sexual victimization in a nonclinical adult sample, *Child Abuse and Neglect*, 12, pp. 51–59.

Briere, J. and Runtz, M. (1993) Child sexual abuse, *Journal of Interpersonal Violence*, 8(3), pp. 312–330.

Briggs, L. and Joyce, P.R. (1997) What determines post-traumatic stress disorder symptomology for survivors of child sexual abuse? *Child Abuse and Neglect*, 21(6), pp. 575–582.

Canton-Cortes, D. and Canton, J. (2010) Coping with child sexual abuse among college students and post-traumatic stress disorder: the role of continuity of abuse and relationship with the perpetrator. *Child Abuse & Neglect*, 34, pp. 496–506.

Carter, J.C., Bewell, C., Blackmore, E. and Woodside, D.B. (2006) The impact of childhood sexual abuse in anorexia nervosa, *Child Abuse and Neglect*, 30(3), pp. 257–269.

Cawson, P., Wattam, C., Brooker, C. and Kelly, G. (2000) *Child Maltreatment in the United Kingdom: A Study of the Prevalence of Child Abuse and Neglect*. London: NSPCC.

Chaffin, M., Silvsky, J.F. and Vaughn, C. (2005) Temporal concordance of anxiety disorders and child sexual abuse: implications for direct versus artifactual effects of sexual abuse, *Journal of Clinical Child & Adolescent Psychology*, 34(2), pp. 210–222.

Cheavens, J.S., Zachary Rosenthal, M., Daughters, S.B., Nowak, J., Kosson, D., Lynch, T.R. and Lejuez, C.W. (2005) An analogue investigation of the relationships among perceived parental criticism, negative affect, and borderline personality disorder features: the role of thought suppression, *Behaviour Research and Therapy*, 43, pp. 257–268.

Chen, L.P., Murad, M.H., Paras, M.L., Colbenson, K.M., Sattler, A.L., Goranson, E.N., Elamin, M.B., Seime, R.J., Shinozaki, G., Prokop, L.J. and Zirakzadeh, A. (2010) Sexual abuse and lifetime diagnosis of psychiatric disorders: systematic review and meta-analysis, *Mayo Clinic Proceedings*, 85(7), pp. 618–629.

Chesler, P. (2005) *Women and Madness*. New York: Palgrave Macmillan.

Claussen, A.H. and Crittenden, P.M. (1991) Physical and psychological maltreatment: relations among types of maltreatment, *Child Abuse and Neglect*, 15, pp. 5–18.

Costin, L.B., Karger, H.J. and Stoesz, D. (1996) *The Politics of Child Abuse in America*. New York: Oxford University Press.

Curtis, C. (2006) Sexual abuse and subsequent suicidal behaviour: exacerbating factors and implications for recovery, *Journal of Child Sexual Abuse*, 15(2), pp. 1–21.

Davis, K. and Taylor, B. (2002) Voices from the margins, part 1: narrative accounts of Indigenous family violence, *Contemporary Nursing*, 14, pp. 240–253.

DeKeseredy, W.S. (2011) Feminist contributions to understanding woman abuse: myths, controversies, and realities, *Aggression and Violent Behavior*, 16, pp. 297–302.

Dhaliwal, G.K., Gauzas, L., Antonowicz, D.H. and Ross, R.R. (1996) Adult male survivors of childhood sexual abuse: prevalence, sexual abuse characteristics, and long-term effects, *Clinical Psychology Review*, 16, pp. 619–639.

Dobash, R.P., Dobash, R.E., Wilson, M. and Daly, M. (1992) The myth of symmetry in marital violence, *Social Problems*, 39, pp. 401–421.

Dong, M., Anda, R.F., Felitti, V.J., Dube, S.R., Williamson, D.F., Thompson, T.J., Loo, C.M. and Giles, W.H. (2004). The interrelatedness of multiple forms of childhood abuse, neglect, and household dysfunction, *Child Abuse & Neglect*, 28, pp. 771–784.

Downs, W.R. and Miller, B.A. (1998) Relationships between experiences of parental violence during childhood and women's psychiatric symptomatology, *Journal of Interpersonal Violence*, 13, pp. 438–457.

Faludi, S. (2006) *Backlash: The Undeclared War Against American Women*. New York: Three Rivers Press.

Featherstone, B. (1997) What has gender got to do with it? Exploring physically abusive behaviour towards children, *British Journal of Social Work*, 3, pp. 419–433.

Fischer, S., Stojek, M. and Hartzell, E. (2010) Effects of multiple forms of childhood abuse and adult sexual assault on current eating disorder symptoms, *Eating Behaviours*, 11(3), pp. 190–192.

Fleming, J., Mullen, P.E., Sibthorne, B. and Gammer, G. (1999) The long-term impact of child sexual abuse in Australian women, *Child Abuse & Neglect*, 23(2), pp. 145–159.

Freyd, J.J. (1997) II: violations of power, adaptive blindness and betrayal trauma theory, *Feminism and Psychology*, 7(1), pp. 22–32.

Gavey, N. (2003) Writing the effects of sexual abuse: interrogating the possibilities and pitfalls of using clinical psychology expertise for a critical justice agenda. In P. Reavey and S. Warner (eds), *New Feminist Stories of Child Sexual Abuse: Sexual Scripts and Dangerous Dialogues*. London: Routledge, pp. 187–209.

Glaser, D. (2011) How to deal with emotional abuse and neglect—further development of a conceptual framework (FRAMEA), *Child Abuse & Neglect*, 35, pp. 866–875.

Golding, J.M. (1999) Intimate partner violence as a risk factor for mental disorders: a meta-analysis, *Journal of Family Violence*, 14(2), pp. 99–132.

Haaken, J. (2003) Traumatic revisions: remembering abuse and the politics of revision. In P. Reavey and S. Warner (eds), *New Feminist Stories of Child Sexual Abuse: Sexual Scripts and Dangerous Dialogues*. London: Routledge, pp. 131–147.

Hacking, I. (1988) The sociology of knowledge about child abuse, *Nous*, 22(1), pp. 53–63.

Heise, L.L. (1998) Violence against women: an integrated, ecological framework, *Violence Against Women*, 4, pp. 262–290.

Herman, J.L. (1997) *Trauma and Recovery*. New York: Basic Books.

Herman, J.L. (2000) *Father-Daughter Incest*. Cambridge, MA: Harvard University Press.

Horsfall, J. (1991) The silent participant: Bryan Turner on anorexia nervosa, *Australian and New Zealand Journal of Sociology*, 27(2), pp. 232–234.

Hulme, P.A. and Agrawal, S. (2004) Patterns of childhood sexual abuse characteristics and their relationships to other childhood abuse, *Journal of Interpersonal Violence*, 19(4), pp. 389–405.

Humphreys, C. and Thiara, R. (2003) Mental health and domestic violence: 'I call it symptoms of abuse', *British Journal of Social Work*, 33(2), pp. 209–226.

Itzin, C., Taket, A. and Barter-Godfrey, S. (2010) *Domestic and Sexual Violence and Abuse: Tackling the Health and Mental Health Effects*. Abingdon: Routledge.

Johnson, J.G., Cohen, P., Brown, J., Smailes, E.M. and Bernstein, D.P. (1999) Childhood maltreatment increases risk for personality disorders during early adulthood, *Journal of the American Medical Association*, 56(7), pp. 600–606.

Johnson, M. and Ferraro, K. (2000) Research on domestic violence in the 1990s: making distinctions. *Journal of Marriage and the Family*, 62, pp. 948–963.

Jones, K.W. (1998) 'Mother made me do it': mother-blaming and the women of child guidance. In M. Ladd-Taylor and L. Umansky (eds), *'Bad' Mothers: The Politics of Blame in Twentieth Century America*. New York: New York University Press, pp. 99–125.

Kennedy, M.A., Ip, K., Samra, J. and Gorzalka, B.B. (2007) The role of childhood emotional abuse in disordered eating, *Journal of Emotional Abuse*, 7(1), pp. 17–36.

Kent, A., Waller, G. and Dagnan, D. (1999) A greater role of emotional than physical or sexual abuse in predicting disordered eating attitudes: the role of mediating variables, *International Journal of Eating Disorders*, 25(2), pp. 159–167.

Laing, L. (1999) A different balance altogether? Incest offenders in treatment. In J. Breckenridge and L. Laing (eds), *Challenging Silence: Innovative Responses to Sexual and Domestic Violence*. Sydney: Allen & Unwin, pp. 137–152.

Laing, L. and Toivonen, C. (2010) *Evaluation of the Domestic Violence and Mental Health Pilot Project*. Faculty of Education and Social Work, University of Sydney.

Lamb, S. (1999) Constructing the victim: popular images and lasting labels. In S. Lamb (ed.), *New Versions of Victims: Feminist Struggle with the Concept*. New York and London: New York University Press, pp. 108–138.

Leskin, G.A. and Sheikh, J.I. (2002) Lifetime trauma history and panic disorder: findings from the National Comorbidity Survey, *Anxiety Disorders*, 16, pp. 599–603.

Levett, A. (2003) Problems of cultural imperialism in the study of child sexual abuse. In P. Reavey and S. Warner (eds), *New Feminist Stories of Child Sexual Abuse: Sexual Scripts and Dangerous Dialogues*. London: Routledge, pp. 52–76.

McCauley, J.M., Kern, D.E., Kolodner, K., Dill, L., Schroeder, A.F., DeChant, H.K., Ryden, J., Bass, E.B. and Derogatis, L.R. (1995) The 'battering syndrome': prevalence and clinical characteristics of domestic violence in primary care internal medicine practices, *Annals of Internal Medicine*, 123(10), pp. 737–746.

May-Chahal, C. (2006) Gender and child maltreatment: the evidence base, *Social Work and Society*, 4(1), pp. 53–68.

Mennen, F.E. and Meadow, D. (1995) The relationship of abuse characteristics to symptoms in sexually abused girls, *Journal of Interpersonal Violence*, 10, pp. 259–274.

Messman-Moore, T.L. and Garrigus, A.S. (2007) The association of child abuse and eating disorder symptomatology: the importance of multiple forms of abuse and revictimization, *Journal of Aggression, Maltreatment & Trauma*, 14(3), pp. 51–72.

Moran, P.M., Bifulco, A., Ball, C., Jacobs, C. and Benaim, K. (2002) Exploring psychological abuse in childhood: I. Developing a new interview scale, *Bulletin of the Menninger Clinic*, 66(3), pp. 213–240.

Mullen, P.E., Martin, J.L., Anderson, S.E., Romans, S.E. and Herbison, G.P. (1996) Long-term impact of the physical, emotional and sexual abuse of children: a community study, *Child Abuse and Neglect*, 20(1), pp. 7–21.

Najman, J.M., Nguyen, M.L.T. and Boyle, F.M. (2007) Sexual abuse in childhood and physical and mental health in adulthood: an Australian population study, *Archives of Sexual Behavior*, 36, pp. 666–675.

National Council to Reduce Violence Against Women and their Children and KPMG Management Consulting (2009) *The Cost of Violence against Women and their Children*. Canberra.

Nurnberg, H.G. and Raskin, M. (1997) Childhood abuse experiences in adult panic disorder, *Medscape Psychiatry and Mental Health e-Journal*, 2(2).

O'Dell, L. (2003) The 'harm' story in child sexual abuse: contested understandings, disputed knowledges. In P. Reavey and S. Warner (eds), *New Feminist Stories of Child Sexual Abuse: Sexual Scripts and Dangerous Dialogues*. London: Routledge, pp. 131–147.

O'Dougherty Wright, M., Crawford, E. and Del Castillo, D. (2009) Childhood emotional maltreatment and later psychological distress among college students: the mediating role of maladaptive schemas, *Child Abuse and Neglect*, 33, pp. 59–68.

Reavey, P. (2003) When past meets present to produce a sexual other: examining professional and everyday narratives of child sexual abuse and sexuality. In P. Reavey and S. Warner (eds), *New Feminist Stories of Child Sexual Abuse: Sexual Scripts and Dangerous Dialogues*. London: Routledge, pp. 148–166.

Reavey, P. and Warner, S. (2003) Introduction. In P. Reavey and S. Warner (eds), *New Feminist Stories of Child Sexual Abuse: Sexual Scripts and Dangerous Dialogues*. London: Routledge, pp. 1–12.

Romano, E. and De Luca, R.V. (2001) Male sexual abuse: a review of effects, abuse characteristics, and links with later psychological functioning, *Aggression and Violent Behaviour*, 6, 55–78.

Romito, P., Molzan Turan, J. and De Marchi, M. (2005) The impact of current and past interpersonal violence on women's mental health, *Social Science & Medicine*, 60, pp. 1717–1727.

Sachs-Ericsson, N., Gayman, M.D., Kendall-Tackett, K., Lloyd, D.A., Medley, A., Collins, N., Corsentino, E. and Sawyer, K. (2010) The long-term impact of childhood abuse on internalizing disorders among older adults: the moderating role of self-esteem, *Aging and Mental Health*, 14(4), pp. 489–501.

Saunders, B.E., Villeponteaux, L.A., Lipovsky, J.A., Kilpatrick, D.G. and Veronen, L.J. (1992) Child sexual assault as a risk factor for mental disorders among women: a community survey, *Journal of Interpersonal Violence*, 7, pp. 189–204.

Scheffer Lindgren, M.S. and Renck, B. (2008) 'It is still so deep-seated, the fear': psychological stress reactions as consequences of intimate partner violence, *Journal of Psychiatric and Mental Health Nursing*, 15(3), pp. 219–228.

Scher, C.D., Forde, D.R., McQuaid, J.R. and Stein, M.B. (2004) Prevalence and demographic correlates of childhood maltreatment in an adult community sample, *Child Abuse and Neglect*, 28(2), 167–180.

Schneider, R., Baumrind, N. and Kimerling, R. (2007) Exposure to child abuse and risk for mental health problems in women, *Violence and Victims*, 22(5), pp. 620–631.

Sedlak, A., Mettenburg, J., Basena, M., Petta, I., McPherson, K., Greene, A. and Li, S. (2010) *Fourth National Incidence Study of Child Abuse and Neglect (NIS-4): Report to Congress*. Washington, DC: U.S. Department of Health and Human Services, Administration for Children and Families.

Shakespeare-Finch, J. and De Dassel, T. (2009) The impact of child sexual abuse on victims/survivors: exploring post-traumatic outcomes as a function of child sexual abuse, *Journal of Child Sexual Abuse*, 18, pp. 623–640.

Spataro, J., Mullen, P.E., Burgess, P.M., Wells, D.L. and Moss, S.A. (2004) Impact of child sexual abuse on mental health: prospective study in males and females, *British Journal of Psychiatry*, 184, pp. 416–421.

Spertus, I.L., Yehuda, R., Wong, C.M., Halligan, S. and Seremetis, S.V. (2003) Childhood emotional abuse and neglect as predictors of psychological and physical symptoms in women presenting to a primary care practice, *Child Abuse and Neglect*, 27, pp. 1247–1258.

Stark, E. (2007) *Coercive Control: How Men Trap Women in Personal Life.* Oxford: Oxford University Press.

Stark, E. and Flitcraft, A. (1996) *Women at Risk: Domestic Violence and Women's Health.* London: Sage.

Stein, M.B., Walker, J.R., Anderson, G., Hazen, A.L., Ross, C.A., Eldridge, G. and Forde, D.L. (1996) Childhood physical and sexual abuse in patients with anxiety disorders and in a community sample, *The American Journal of Psychiatry*, 153(2), pp. 275–277.

Stoltenborgh, M. (2012) The universality of childhood emotional abuse: a meta-analysis of worldwide prevalence, *Journal of Aggression, Maltreatment and Trauma*, 21(8), pp. 870–890.

Stoltenborgh, M., van Ijzendoorn, M.H., Euser, E.M. and Bakermans-Kranenburg, M.J. (2011) A global perspective on child sexual abuse: meta-analysis of prevalence around the world, *Child Maltreatment*, 16, pp. 79–101.

Trickett, P.K., Noll, J.G. and Putnam, F.W. (2011) The impact of sexual abuse on female development: lessons from a multigenerational, longitudinal research study, *Development and Psychopathology*, 23, pp. 453–476.

Tseris, E. (2013) Trauma theory without feminism? Evaluating contemporary understandings of traumatised women, *Affilia: The Journal of Women in Social Work*, 28, pp. 153–164.

United Nations (UN) (1993) *Declaration on the Elimination of Violence against Women.* Available at: http://daccess-dds-ny.un.org/doc/RESOLUTION/GEN/NR0/711/88/IMG/NR071188.pdf?OpenElement, accessed 22 April 2015.

Walby, S. (2004) *The Cost of Domestic Violence.* Women and Equality Unit, UK.

Walby, S., Towers, J. and Francis, B. (2014) Mainstreaming domestic and gender-based violence into sociology and the criminology of violence, *The Sociological Review*, 62(S2), pp. 187–214.

Warner, S. (2009) *Understanding the Effects of Child Sexual Abuse: Feminist Revolutions in Theory, Research and Practice.* London: Routledge.

Warner, S. and Wilkins, T. (2003) Diagnosing distress and reproducing disorder: women, child sexual abuse and 'borderline personality disorder'. In P. Reavey and S. Warner (eds), *New Feminist Stories of Child Sexual Abuse: Sexual Scripts and Dangerous Dialogues.* London: Routledge, pp. 167–186.

World Health Organization (WHO) (2013) *Global and Regional Estimates of Violence against Women: Prevalence and Health Effects of Intimate Partner Violence and Non-Partner Sexual Violence.* Geneva: WHO. Available at: www.who.int/reproductive-health/publications/violence/9789241564625/en/, accessed 22 April 2015.

3   Researching gendered violence, abuse and mental health

In this chapter, I outline my theoretical and methodological approach to under-taking feminist research into gendered violence, abuse and mental health. As noted in Chapter 2, there has been a growing body of post-structural feminist research into gendered abuse and mental health over the past two decades that has been primarily concerned with child sexual abuse. There has also been increasing research by feminist scholars into the impact of domestic violence on mental health, with most of this emanating from a structural feminist tradition. As yet, there has been no feminist consideration of childhood emotional abuse and mental health. The three research studies that form the basis of the rest of this book consider all types of gendered violence and abuse from the perspective that they often occur together and have the greatest impact on mental health when they do. In this chapter, my aim is to outline how I sought to unite a post-structural feminist awareness of the structuring effects of language, fluid subjec-tivities, difference and the constructive aspects of power with structural and material feminist concerns about women's real, lived experiences of mental health problems in social contexts that continue to be framed by gender oppres-sion. There have been calls for some time from feminist theorists, such as Lois McNay (2004), urging feminists to consider both the symbolic and material dimensions of the problems women encounter in their day-to-day lives. This is what I aim to achieve through exploration of the impact of gendered violence and abuse on women's mental health and wellbeing. I will admit, though, that it is no easy task to navigate the intersections between the discursive and the material simultaneously, and I discuss some of the challenges of attempting to do so later.

Travels around feminism: feminist social work and research in mental health

As briefly mentioned in the introductory chapter, my own feminist journey com-menced in the second wave of feminism in the mid-1980s. While the women's movement was probably most active in Australia in the 1970s, it was during the 1980s that it successfully established many dynamic women's services through a highly successful feminist 'infiltration' of government bureaucracies by so-called 'femocrats' (Broom, 1991). These services were arguably at their strongest during the 1980s, and I came into contact with them through my social work studies. My field placements and my initial social work positions were primarily in women's services, including feminist women's health centres, and perhaps for the first time the problems facing women in their day-to-day lives, my own included, started to make at least some sense. I would have to say that up until that time, few of the psychological or sociological theories that I had encountered at university (other than Marxism) seemed to relate to my experiences growing up as a white, Catholic-educated, working-class girl from the far-flung outer suburbs of Adelaide, a middle-sized (and often overlooked) southern Australian city. However, the feminist insight that 'the personal is political' certainly meant something, and was both exciting and a *relief*. For the first time, I encountered the sense that perhaps I was not alone in my struggles with confidence and trying to make my way in the world on the back of an upbringing framed by deep ambivalence about the place and value of women and girls. The idea that there was a commonality to women's problems, including struggles with identity and sense of self, was therefore experienced as enormously liberating personally, but also brought new ways of working that challenged traditional conceptualisations of professional expertise and detachment. While we did not distinguish much between different 'types' of feminism as health and community workers during this time, our approach was probably most accurately described as a mix of structuralist feminism, with conceptions of patriarchy and socio-economic gender and class inequalities at its centre, liberal feminist ideas of choice and rights, and the appropriation of certain concepts from social psychology that suited our purposes, such as the constructs of self-esteem, self-assertion and cognitive-behavioural learning theories. We undertook counselling based on principles of empowerment and partnership; group work based on connecting women with each other rather than with professionals; and community development that sought to address alongside local women some of the structural elements of social disadvantage in their lives, such as lack of child-care, based on the public health idea that 'upstream' action was preventive of later 'downstream' health problems (Kingdon, 1995).

One of the main issues we confronted in our work was gendered violence and abuse, and we worked with women from a diversity of class and cultural backgrounds who were experiencing these problems. Often, the women did not divulge sexual abuse histories until they felt safe, and this might be weeks or months after counselling or groups had commenced. Child sexual abuse had not yet gained the public or professional attention it now receives and I therefore learned through listening directly to the women how common and hidden this form of abuse was. At the time, I did not have specific ways of working with women who had been sexually abused, but I could well see that these experiences were distressing for them, and I focused on empathic listening, helping them see it was not their fault and confidence-building. Domestic violence was better recognised at the time, and the emphasis of our work was focused on helping women leave safely because we believed, perhaps simplistically and naively, that self-esteem would improve and anxiety would lessen if women got away from their abusive partners and became independent. However, there was another type of abuse that women commonly raised but for which there was no name at the time: childhood emotional abuse. Some women traced their struggles with self-esteem and self-assertion to oppressive and controlling practices in their families of origin: again, my approach focused on helping women see they were not to blame and on confidence-building. While these were exciting days in the women's health movement, the feminist terrain was shifting towards the end of the 1980s and into the early 1990s, with the emergence of identity politics.

Into the 1990s, there was a splintering of feminist interests in Australia, just as in other Western countries (also see Warner, 2009, for an account of this from a UK perspective). This was triggered by criticisms from black women, women from other cultural groups and lesbian women that white, heterosexual, Western feminism did not necessarily speak to their needs or issues (McNay, 1992; Stanley and Wise, 1990). Over the past three decades, black women in particular have pointed out that it is only for privileged, white Western women that gender is the central form of oppression, and that dominant forms of feminism generalise these experiences to all women (McNay, 1992). Thus, power differences *between* women became the focus in recognition that these have far-reaching implications for the struggle against gender oppression (McNay, 1992). While such criticisms were and are valid, it often became necessary within the feminist movement and women's services to identify oneself by race or class, or by sexuality, and a wider feminist concern with common interests was less in evidence. Not dissimilarly to Sam Warner's experiences in the UK (Warner, 2009), I also found my passion for redressing gender inequalities waning a little during this period as feminism became increasingly fraught and fragmented. At the same time, backlash politics gained ground (Faludi, 2006) alongside the erroneous belief that the gender war had been won and that women had achieved equality (Reavey and Warner, 2003). Certainly, public awareness of domestic violence seemed muted during this period, although attention to child sexual abuse had grown exponentially. I worked in women's health services during this time, too, right when the so-called 'memory wars' were in full force. We continued to work with many women who had experienced child sexual abuse, but the presentation among a minority had changed so that satanic ritual abuse and multiple personality disorders were sometimes described (although not often), while a small number of women believed or suspected they were abused but had no memory of it. Such cases proved to be divisive because some feminist practitioners urged that the women's stories must always be believed and taken at face value, while others felt a level of wariness about the more extreme accounts (see Haaken, 2003, for an insightful discussion about how expectations that women's accounts of abuse be transparent reflections of external events strips them of their complexity and denies imagination, symbolisation and social construction in accounting for distressing experiences). A new, highly political approach to therapy was also gaining ground in Australia and elsewhere at this time: narrative therapy. Michael White's Dulwich Centre was, and continues to be, based in Adelaide and many local feminist practitioners such as myself, as well as others from around Australia and the world, gained training here in its principles and methods. However, as noted in the previous chapter, the more political aspects of feminist activism continued to be in little evidence throughout this period and the women's health movement and its political insights were becoming lost as mainstream psychological and medical services became increasingly involved in the provision of mental health services to abused women, but without the political insights of feminism (see also Armstrong, 1994; Lamb, 1999; O'Dell, 2003; Warner, 2009).

It was in the mid-1990s that I moved into academia to pursue my interests in gender and mental health further. This shift was in part motivated by a level of frustration with an increasingly conservative approach to women's mental health struggles, particularly the rise in biological models of mental illness (Ussher, 2010). This heralded another watershed moment in my travels around feminism with the discovery of post-structuralism, where I came face-to-face all at once with the seismic shifts that had been occurring within feminist academia, as well as the humanities and social sciences more generally, during the intervening ten years while I had been in the practice field. Up until that time, my sole engagement with post-structuralism had been through narrative therapy. I only really began to grasp the implications of post-structural thought in a deeper, more meaningful way when I embarked on my doctoral studies, which involved an exploration of the gendered discourses used in the explanation, treatment and prevention of eating disorders, a particularly gendered mental health problem. A fellow PhD candidate described to me how she became quite frightened when she first grasped the post-structural idea that social reality is constructed through language and discourse, because this meant there were no certainties and everything was potentially up for question. I had a similar reaction: while I had encountered other philosophical thought during my studies that questioned received reality, it was post-structuralism that offered a more profound and complex insight into the constructive effects of language, the connections between knowledge and power, and the multiple, fluid nature of subjectivity (Foucault, 1972, 1977a, 1977b). Unsurprisingly, I suppose, along with this came a level of ontological insecurity. However, I never threw out the understanding that discourse is framed by, and embedded within, structures of inequality and that there are dominant discourses that reflect vested interests. Like many other feminists in social work and other disciplines concerned with social change, I continue to understand my post-structural feminist approach as the meeting of two theoretical traditions – post-structuralism and feminism – and eschewed the more extreme relativism of the post-modern (also see Warner, 2009; Wendt and Zannettino, 2015). As such, I continue to grapple with the challenge of how to attend more fulsomely to the discursive, symbolic dimensions of women's lives, their material dimensions and the structural inequalities that frame them. As noted in the introduction, in Australia as well as other countries both developed and developing, violence against women has recently become the most prominent battleground for the contemporary feminist movement, so attempting to bridge the gap between the discursive and the material through examination of gendered violence and mental health is hopefully timely and fruitful, both academically and in terms of action.

Feminist theoretical approaches to gendered violence and mental health

Post-structural feminism

'Post-structuralism' refers to the philosophical movement that is associated with the writings on language, discourse and texts produced initially by French cultural analysts such as Derrida, Lyotard and Foucault in the late 1960s, 1970s and 1980s (Parker, 1992). Post-structural feminism is crucial to the research reported in this book because it brings an awareness that 'concepts such as truth are subject to a wide range of interpretations that depend on who is speaking and the position they are speaking from' (Reavey and Warner, 2003: 1). Medical and psychological discourses are powerful and dominant in the mental health arena, and a post-structural feminist perspective is critically important in helping to deconstruct and understand the effects of these, as well as identify their unspoken gender assumptions. Post-structural feminism is also vital for exploring and revealing the diversity of understandings and experiences of gendered violence and abuse (Reavey and Warner, 2003; Warner, 2009; Wendt and Zannettino, 2015), including resistance to dominant, pathologising discourses of blame and victimhood. Much of the plethora of psycho-medical research into gendered violence, abuse and mental health seeks to identify cause and delineate the nature of psychopathology from within a positivist, medico-scientific epistemological paradigm, based on the assumption that mental health problems constitute real, distinct entities that can be quantified, known and treated in an objective sense. This affects women's experiences of mental health problems in contexts of abuse in multiple ways in that the knowledge applied to their distress, and the associated interventions in which they participate, become imbricated in their actual experiences of distress. This alludes to the role of the human sciences, and the associated practice disciplines, in constructing the very 'conditions' they seek to quantify, explain and treat (Parker *et al.*, 1995).

The research studies into gendered violence, abuse and mental health that form the basis for this book draw, among other things, on the post-structural ideas of the French philosopher, Michel Foucault. Foucault emphasised the role of language in the discursive production of reality, where language is comprised of historically specific discourses described as 'practices that systematically form the objects of which they speak' (Foucault, 1972: 49). Thus, for Foucault, discourse does not simply reflect social reality, but is constitutive of it (Henriques *et al.*, 1984; Parker, 1992; Burman and Parker, 1993). This is a radically different view of language as bringing objects into meaning, rather than conveying a meaning that precedes language (Foucault, 1977b). The idea that discursive practices form the objects of which they speak extends to a concern with how individual subjects are constructed in discourse (Parker, 1992; Burman and Parker, 1993). Thus, language is understood as 'the place where actual and possible forms of social organisation and their likely social and political consequences are defined and contested ... it is also the place where our sense of ourselves, our subjectivity, is constructed' (Weedon, 1987: 21).

Subjectivity is seen as produced in a range of discursive practices and the meanings of these are understood as 'a site of struggle over power' (Weedon, 1987: 21). Furthermore, the subject positions produced through discursive practices are multiple, shifting and often contradictory, challenging the humanist assumption of a fixed and stable self (Parker, 1992). The notion that discursive practices involve a struggle over power is based on the idea that power and knowledge are intrinsically linked and 'directly imply one another' (Foucault, 1977a: 27). Thus, 'there is no power relation without the correlative constitution of a field of knowledge, nor any knowledge that does not presuppose and constitute at the same time power relations' (Foucault, 1977a: 27).

For Foucault, then, discursive practices are intrinsically tied up with power and knowledge, and the point at which discourse emerges is synonymous with the production of truth (Foucault, 1982). Thus, 'ways of knowing are equated with ways of exercising power over individuals', where disciplinary power is understood to be written on the body and soul of the individual (Sawicki, 1991: 22). The discursive practices that constitute the professional fields of gendered violence and of mental health can therefore be understood as involving power relations, where truth and subjectivity are at stake.

Foucault's work also involves a focus on the body as discursively produced through historically specific power relations, rather than as a pre-existent or natural entity (McNay, 1992). Foucault understands the body to be 'produced through power', and as a historically specific and 'cultural rather than a natural entity', and while Foucault does not elide the corporeality of the body, his perspective represents a radical departure from conventional and scientific assumptions about the body (McNay, 1992: 3). Foucault describes the way in which discourse becomes inscribed on the body, producing subjected and practised 'docile' bodies reflective of, and constitutive of, wider social relations (Foucault, 1977a: 138). This notion of the body as caught up in wider power relations is important because it offers the potential for understanding the impact of gendered violence and abuse on women's bodies – their emotions and their mental and physical wellbeing – as constitutive of gender discourses and wider gender power relations rather than only of 'sickness' and 'pathology'. While Foucault examines the disciplinary effects of power on subjectivity and the body, his view of power does not involve a notion of a universal, sovereign entity, though. Rather, power is conceived of as diffuse, and is exercised rather than possessed (Sawicki, 1991), while power relations are decentred (Foucault, 1978). Furthermore, while power is understood as operating through discourse to regulate and discipline individuals (Foucault, 1977a), it is also understood to be productive and positive, not merely repressive and negative, and as producing resistance to its disciplinary effects (Foucault, 1978; McNay, 1992). Foucault (1980) defined resistance as arising where the operation of power is most repressive, and this idea is therefore closely linked with the notion of productive power (McNay, 1992). Thus, I do not assume that women are the mere docile bodies or passive subjects of either gendered violence or of mental health intervention. Rather, women are actively involved in the processes of subjectification, including the potential to resist the subjectivities they impose (Foucault, 1978, 1988). Thus, while I am concerned with examining the oppressive, negative effects of gendered violence on women's wellbeing, this is tempered by an awareness that women's experiences are not wholly reducible to the oppressive effects of power.

Feminists have drawn on post-structural theory to emphasise the ways in which gender inequalities are reproduced in the structuring of explanations of women through historical, social and political discourse (for example, Weedon, 1987; Sawicki, 1991; McNay, 1992; Butler, 1993). Thus, feminist engagement with post-structuralism has extended understandings of the way bodies and subjectivities are produced in discourse by acknowledging the 'gendered character' of many of the disciplinary techniques that circumscribe the female body (McNay, 1992: 11). Feminist analyses have shown in particular that psychological theory, which informs much of contemporary psychiatry, psychology and other disciplines involved in the treatment of 'mental illness', is itself intrinsically gendered. Western thought is underpinned by a series of core dichotomies, in particular, the association of 'male' with reason, culture, the universal and the public, and 'female' with the irrational, emotion, the physical, nature, the particular and private (Jaggar, 1989: Lloyd, 1989). These ideas are also linked to Cartesian dualism, where the mind is seen as synonymous with the self and superior to the physical body (Lloyd, 1989). These assumptions also structure psychological knowledge, so that the idealised model of the 'thinking, reasoning individual' is a model of man, made possible by the subordinate positioning of women in gender power relations that result in 'male-defined criteria of normality' (Burman *et al.*, 1996: 3). Gendered ideas about 'mental health' have particular effects within contemporary mental health care practice more generally, most clearly illustrated in a now famous study conducted in the 1970s by Broverman *et al.* (1972). Mental health clinicians were shown to perceive socially acceptable 'feminine' characteristics, such as dependency and emotionality, as conflicting with notions of mental healthiness because they are at odds with notions of instrumentality and adulthood (Broverman *et al.*, 1972). Conversely, 'masculine' characteristics were unproblematically understood as marks of mental health in men (Broverman *et al.*, 1972). Thus, notions of mental health in women are inherently conflicted and contradictory because they operate around 'a double standard of mental health' (Chesler, 2005: xxi) and contemporary feminists, myself included, have continued to demonstrate the operation of this double standard in current mental health practices (for example, Malson, 1998; Moulding, 2003, 2006; Wirth-Cauchon, 2001).

Some feminist theorists have utilised the later ideas of Foucault to show that dominant constructions of gender are oppressive but do not completely determine women's experiences and actions (for example, McNay, 1992; Probyn, 1993). Feminist theorists have also drawn on a range of other ideas to elaborate that discourse is not completely determining. Perhaps most well-known is Judith Butler's idea of gender as 'performative', which has provided a way of thinking about gender identity not as entirely determined or constructed, but as 'a regularised and constrained reiteration of norms' (Butler, 1993: 94–95). Butler (1993) emphasises the temporal nature of performativity, where 'sex is both produced and destabilized in the course of reiteration' (Butler, 1993: 10). The reiteration of sexual norms is seen as indicative of their instability, and of the possibility for change through the creation of 'a potentially productive crisis' (Butler, 1993: 10) and the 're-signification of the symbolic domain' (Butler, 1993: 22), leaving space for the exercise of individual agency.

Post-structural feminists have made important contributions to understanding the gendered assumptions underpinning knowledge and practice in relation to mental health (for example, Malson, 1998; Wirth-Cauchon, 2001; Ussher, 1991, 2010) and mental health in the context of abuse, specifically child sexual abuse (Reavey and Warner, 2003; Warner, 2009). There has been less post-structural feminist engagement with the issue of domestic violence outside of the work of my colleagues, Sarah Wendt and Lana Zannettino (2015), and, as noted earlier, much of the feminist research in this area has been more structuralist with only limited feminist attention to domestic violence and mental health. Gendered violence and abuse are among the most extreme manifestations of the oppression of women and children in patriarchal societies (Walby, 1990). There is general agreement among feminist researchers, practitioners and activists of all feminist persuasions that gender inequalities both enable and reproduce gendered violence and abuse, and that women and children are far and away its most likely victims while men are the most likely perpetrators (for example, Itzin *et al.*, 2010; Reavey and Warner, 2003; Walby, 1990; Walby *et al.*, 2014; Warner, 2009). Of course language remains critical to our understandings and experiences of violence and abuse, just as it does to mental health, but language is embedded within gender and other social power relations of privilege and disadvantage. Post-structural feminist research into gendered abuse and mental health acknowledges wider gender power inequalities and is careful to emphasise that both abuse and the distress it causes are real (for example, Reavey and Warner, 2003; Warner, 2009). While post-structural feminist approaches to the study of gendered violence and abuse includes acknowledgement of wider gender power relations and Enlightenment ideas of social transformation and change, I want to be more explicit than this about the gender inequalities that discourse is embedded within, and the material impact of gendered violence and abuse on mental health and wellbeing. As such, I adopt McNay's (2004) concept of situated inter-subjectivity, which attends to both discourse and to material lived experience, including the often overlooked emotional dimensions of gendered violence and abuse.

Situated intersubjectivity: navigating the discursive and the material

The concept of situated intersubjectivity outlined by McNay (2004) understands the discursive aspects of identity and everyday intersubjective material power relations as inherently intertwined. McNay (2004) argues that one of the key debates in contemporary feminist theory has been 'that between material and cultural feminists about how to conceptualise the nature of gender oppression and, by implication, the possibilities for change' (McNay, 2004: 172). Drawing on Nancy Fraser (2000), she argues further that this has created a raft of 'false antitheses', where economic analyses of oppression are opposed to discursive analyses of identity. McNay (2004) suggests that this has hindered more constructive examination of how cultural and material feminisms might be combined, and she offers up the concept of situated intersubjectivity as a way forward:

> I argue that situated intersubjectivity may serve as a way of more securely integrating cultural feminist work on the linguistic construction of gender identity with an analysis of power relations suggested by materialist feminism. In sum, the idea of intersubjectivity provides a category through which the intertwinement of symbolic and material power relations can begin to be thought.
>
> (McNay, 2004: 172)

Cultural feminism developed from the 'linguistic turn' brought by post-structural theory and attempted to overcome what were seen as rigid, overly fixed and simplified concepts of patriarchy and oppression (McNay, 2004). However, while post-structural feminist concepts such as discourse and performativity have been very influential, McNay (2004) argues that the 'pendulum seems to have come full circle' through the criticism that 'all issues of gender oppression are treated in the narrow terms of positionality within language' in post-structural theories (p. 173). She argues that a reduction of everything to language does not provide or enable a differentiated analysis of power relations to explore new forms of gender autonomy and dependence (McNay, 2004). For example, post-structural feminist research into child sexual abuse sometimes professes to approach knowledge as if all claims are equivalent, and this relativism can play down identification of dominant discourses and associated gender power relations. This research can also remain at an abstract, discursive level of explanation to the exclusion of attention to the material impact of abuse on women and their lives. McNay (2004) also points out how post-structural theory, such as Butler's (1993) performativity, 'remains caught within a privatized and individualistic conception of activity whose radical political status is open to question in so far as it is complicit with, rather than disruptive of, capitalism' (p. 173). She argues that by absorbing society into language alone, cultural feminists fail to see the 'the complex and uneven ways in which gender inequalities are produced', including underestimating how intractable some forms of oppression are and overestimating how much change can be brought through cultural identity politics (p. 174).

Post-structural feminist research into child sexual abuse and mental health can also reflect this problem by prioritising individual and conceptual/symbolic change over structural change, yet these are arguably tied together and, I argue, both are required simultaneously.

Material feminists are therefore more cautious about change, arguing that it is gradual and complicated, with new forms of autonomy very often coinciding with new types of subordination and dependency (McNay, 2004). McNay (2004) draws attention to Sylvia Walby's observation that 'while gender relations could potentially take an infinite number of forms, in actuality there are some widely repeated features' (Walby, 1990: 16). This observation undoubtedly has relevance to the study of gendered violence and abuse: it is widely accepted that there has been little or no decline in the rates of gendered violence, including in developed countries, in spite of other changes in opportunities for women (WHO, 2013). Not dissimilarly, child sexual abuse shows no signs of having reduced since its 're-discovery' in the 1970s, in spite of increased awareness of children's rights, at least in Western countries, and some shifts in gender relations. Gender ideologies, identities and norms are clearly relevant to this, but material feminists argue that violence against women also rests on broader forms of patriarchal control. In theorising violence against women, Walby (1990) argues that while male violence involves the use of power over women in its own right, it is also 'importantly shaped as a result of patriarchal control over women in other areas' (p. 143). Walby (2006) defines patriarchy as 'a social system of gender relations in which there is gender inequality', where women are generally disadvantaged compared to men (p. 121). She particularly draws attention to how gender inequality is interrelated, with causal connections between the different domains and male-perpetrated violence one such domain (Walby, 2006). Thus, there are clearly structural dimensions to gendered violence and abuse. In drawing attention to the links between male violence, abuse and patriarchal control, Walby (1990) particularly emphasises the historical (and largely continuing) failure of the state to adequately intervene to name male violence and abuse against women and children as criminal, and its concomitant failure to properly provide the means for women (and children) to escape dependence on violent men (Walby, 1990).

Materialist feminism therefore draws attention to the reproduction of gender power relations, and the links to socio-economic and state structures, in violence against women and children. However, McNay (2004) also argues that this, in turn, can be at the expense of other kinds of social and cultural experience. What is lost, she argues, is a 'hermeneutic notion of self and a coherent account of subjectivity and agency through which the daily experiences of economic, social and cultural oppression might be conceived of as co-extensive rather than crudely determining of each other' (McNay, 2004: 175). I argue that this is particularly pertinent to the study of gendered violence, abuse and mental health. Without feminist ways of theorising and understanding the thinking, feeling, acting subject and their gendered positioning, we are left with psycho-medical notions of damaged selves and victimhood. Indeed, materialist feminism has not particularly applied itself to the field of gender and mental health, or to challenging the dominance of psycho-medical theories and practices. It is post-structural feminists who have stepped into this space and developed sophisticated insights into the nature of women's distress that challenge psychological and medical discourses, and their claims to objectivity and gender neutrality. Thus, as is argued by McNay (2004), the concept of situated intersubjectivity is a useful corrective to the individualising tendencies of post-structuralism, because it explicitly embeds the subject in social relations and also counteracts a materialist tendency to prioritise structures over experience by emphasising intention and agency on the part of the subject. She argues further that 'the idea of intersubjectivity contains within itself a way of connecting experience to the power relations that sustain and structure it' (McNay, 2004: 177). Situated intersubjectivity therefore seems a particularly appropriate theoretical frame for researching women's understandings and experiences of emotional distress in the context of violent and abusive social relations of gender, as well as the pathways women find out of this distress.

In addition to the concept of situated intersubjectivity and its emphasis on the entwinement of the symbolic and material, I specifically situate women's sense of themselves and their emotional distress in *relationships*. Althusser (1971; Warner, 2009) proposed the concept of 'interpellation', arguing that a subject is interpellated when 's/he recognises him/herself in the symbolic structures of society' (McNay, 2008: 174). Thus, the individual is interpellated through their imaginary relationship with their social network (Warner, 2009), but ideology functions such that individuals disavow that their sense of themselves is located in social processes of identification in their everyday lives (McNay, 2008; Warner, 2009). Warner (2009) argues further that child sexual abuse naturalises certain forms of subjectivity and that the operations of power within this remain hidden from those who are abused. Taking this further, then, the abused child comes to recognise themselves as a certain kind of individual – for example, as 'blameworthy', 'bad' and 'mad' – and in many respects, dominant psycho-medical discourses of mental illness do not particularly challenge this: in fact they sometimes reinforce such identities. This concept of self-in-relationship emerges as central across all of the studies discussed in following chapters, and is taken up further in discussion of practice responses to gendered violence and abuse in Chapter 8.

Centring the emotional dimensions of gendered violence and abuse

In addition to the theoretical considerations above, the research presented in this book pays particular attention to the place of emotion in women's accounts of gendered violence, abuse and mental health. During the 1990s, the social sciences encountered what has been referred to as 'the affective turn', which suggested that in order to theorise the social, it is necessary to attend to affect, or emotion (Clough and Halley, 2007). This reflected a growing interest in the ways that cultural, political and economic transformations were changing the social realm, particularly affect, understood as bodily forces which influence individual capacity to interact with others (Clough and Halley, 2007). My interest in the emotional dimensions of gendered violence and abuse perhaps most clearly reflects the interconnections between the discursive and the more material realist dimensions of women's experiences of mental health problems in contexts of violence and abuse.

Much psychological research treats emotion as the by-product or cause of pathology. Herman (1997) specifically implores researchers and practitioners to attend more fulsomely to the emotional dimensions of the psychological distress experienced by women who have been abused, arguing that this has often been overlooked. However, I take a feminist and sociological view of emotion as constituted in the intersubjective dynamics between individuals (Crawford *et al.*, 1992: 9) and as representing 'the domain of the repressed that betrays the structure of regulation' (Burman *et al.*, 1996: 13). I therefore argue that emotion has much to tell us about experiences of oppression, particularly highly subjugated and silenced forms such as gendered violence and abuse as well as mental illness. I specifically draw on Williams' (1977) theory of structures of feeling, which understands emotion as a social experience rather than a private and isolating one, and re-theorises the relationship between thought and feeling, which are universally separated in psychological theory, as 'not feeling against thought, but thought as felt and feeling as thought' (Williams, 1977: 132). Within such a conceptualisation, emotion becomes meaningful and potentially reflective of a particular socio-historical period and its concerns, rather than a privatised experience reflective only of individual 'pathology'.

Overviewing the three studies

The three research studies into gendered violence, abuse and mental health that form the basis of exploration and discussion in the rest of the book draw on a total of 43 individual interviews and qualitative responses from 613 women to an online survey. The first study is explored in Chapter 4 and involved interviews with women and men who had experienced childhood emotional abuse. As noted, no studies have specifically considered the gendered dimensions and dynamics of child emotional abuse, nor those of race and class. This study was concerned with elaborating the social discourses and practices in women's and men's narratives and experiences of childhood emotional abuse, the emotions related to these and the relationship of these to wider gender and other social inequalities. The second study, which is considered in Chapters 4 and 5, involved interviews with women who had experienced eating disorders, and I focus particularly on the narratives of those women who identified that they had experienced eating disorders in contexts of abuse. This study aimed to explore how women explain the emergence of an eating disorder in their lives over time in relation to abuse, and particularly attended to the meanings of eating disorder symptoms in contexts of abuse, and their role in managing abuse-related emotion. The first two studies therefore focused on childhood abuse and mental health. The third research study focused on domestic violence and mental health, and is the focus of Chapter 6. This research is a large mixed methods study involving a national, community-based online survey and qualitative life history interviews with women who have experienced domestic violence. The survey involved both quantitative and qualitative questions about the impact of domestic violence on women's lives. This study is still continuing and is not mine alone: it is being conducted by a team of colleagues, including myself, from the University of South Australia and Curtin University in Western Australia.[1] The wider study is concerned with the impact of domestic violence on women's citizenship, and looks not only at mental health but also at employment and housing, with all three domains understood to be key dimensions of citizenship. My colleagues have kindly agreed to allow me to draw on the mental health data for this book and, as such, some of the interpretations and conclusions drawn here should not be assumed to be those of the team as a whole. The analysis I present from this study focuses specifically on the ways women constructed the impact of domestic violence on mental health. Lastly, all three studies also attended to experiences of recovery from abuse-related mental health problems, and this aspect of the narratives is considered in Chapter 7 as part of exploring the prospects for feminist-informed practice in this area.

Interviewing and ethical considerations

Of particular concern to feminist researchers is the issue of power relations between the researcher and the research participant (Stanley and Wise, 1990; Grbich, 1999). One of the most central principles of a feminist approach to research is to attempt a non-exploitative, egalitarian and emancipatory relationship between the researcher and the researched (Grbich, 1999). Oakley (1981), for example, argues that traditional approaches to social research interviews are based on a masculinist approach, emphasising a one-way flow of information, the objectification of the research participant, a supposedly detached and objective researcher and the impersonal nature of interaction between the researcher and the researched. These are at odds with a feminist perspective emphasising the validation of women's subjective experiences (Oakley, 1981), the equalising of relations between researcher and researched (Grbich, 1999) and in-depth interview methods that are dialogic rather than one-directional (Sarantakos, 2012). I very much approached the interviews informed by these feminist principles, as did my colleagues who also undertook interviews in the domestic violence study. While the interviews are probably best described as semi-structured because a series of interview questions was developed for each study, I did not impose a structure and allowed participants to tell me their stories in the way that seemed to best serve them. As such, some participants offered relatively chronological accounts while others preferred to shift back and forwards across time according to topics they were covering. I placed a real emphasis on careful listening and I tried to pick up on issues that seemed especially relevant to participants, but also those that were important to me in the sense that they alluded to the gendered dimensions of experience. The interviews were dialogic in the sense that at times they became conversations where we both considered the meanings of the account and its implications. Moreover, because individuals were often talking about distressing experiences and sometimes became upset, it was critical to be empathic and to actively demonstrate this in my responses to participants.

The interviews for the three studies ran for between one and two hours and were conducted either in university staff offices, community services or in the women's homes. In a couple of instances, participants in the childhood emotional abuse study were interviewed twice because they needed and wanted additional time to cover all the issues they thought important: a number of interviewees for this study had never accounted their experiences of abuse before. The interviews were digitally recorded and transcribed verbatim. Details about recruitment and the samples for all three studies are provided in subsequent chapters. The three studies were approved by the University of South Australia Human Research Ethics Committee, and informed written consent was obtained from participants prior to participation.

Analysis of interview and survey data

The data was analysed through a combination of thematic analysis and narrative-discursive analysis. The thematic analysis was informed by a post-structural feminist perspective that attended inductively to the diversity of ideas individuals drew on to explain their experiences, as well as a material feminist engagement with the lived reality of those experiences, particularly the emotions, and the wider gender power relations framing them (Braun and Clarke, 2006). I chose to conduct a narrative-discursive analysis because this approach unites attention to discourse and multiple identities with the more continuous aspects of lived identity over time (Taylor and Littleton, 2006: 25) and their historical and social contexts (Riessman, 2008; Taylor and Littleton, 2006). Mental health problems associated with childhood abuse in particular usually emerge over many years so there are continuous elements to the subjectivities involved, while many women's experiences of domestic violence and emotional distress also occurred over lengthy periods of time. As noted earlier, I also attended to the emotional dimensions of experience as part of the analysis undertaken in all three studies. I will now describe the steps in the data analysis in a little more detail, starting with thematic analysis, followed by narrative analysis and then discourse analysis.

All three studies included an initial thematic analysis to identify key themes across the interview data as the first step in the process of analysis (Braun and Clarke, 2006). This involved initial axial coding of the main themes in each data set, followed by more detailed selective coding of specific sub-themes and the relationships between them (Sarantakos, 2012). This initial thematic categorisation was conducted within and across each data set, meaning thematic material was 'chunked' together from across the interviews in each of the studies, but the data was not combined into one large data set. This is because the three studies were distinctive from each other, even though thematic analysis did identify some broad thematic similarities. For example, I identified a large category of talk in all three studies about the impact of violence and abuse on sense of self and identity. Terms employed by participants that denoted this category included talk about 'identity', finding a 'true self', 'losing a sense of oneself' or having 'no sense of self'. I used the electronic data analysis package, NVivo, for the process of thematic categorisation, but only as a data manager, not for actual analysis.

It has been widely noted that when individuals describe themselves and their lives, they tend to automatically offer a narrative – a story – with a beginning, middle and end, and events organised temporally within (Taylor, 2006). Thus, narrators typically 'look back on and recount lives that are located in particular times and places' which is both personal and reflects broader social dynamics (Riessman, 2008: 7). However, biographies or life histories need not construct a linear, single narrative (Bryant and Hoon, 2006), but can also involve conflicted, shifting and complex histories (Reay, 1997). Moreover, structured, temporally organised narratives are social constructions in themselves (Mishler, 1997) and not all narratives are organised in this way (Riessman, 2008). In particular, the experience of illness in an individual's life often disrupts the life narrative (Frank, 1995), while non-white and less educated groups do not necessarily participate in Western, culturally dominant narrative forms (Riessman, 2008). For the narrative analysis, I mainly drew on Riessman's (2008) account of the processes that can be employed. Riessman's (2008) explanation of narrative analysis is not a 'how to' manual, but rather a thoughtful account, using exemplars, of the ways that researchers have used narrative analysis in the human sciences. Narrative analysis refers to a group of methods for analysing texts that deal with 'the storied form' (Riessman, 2008: 11), with a focus on 'particular actors, in particular social places, at particular social times' (Abbott, 1992: 428, cited in Riessman, 2008: 11). The focus of narrative analysis is on how participants assemble and sequence events through language in order to communicate meaning (Riessman, 2008). However, narrative analysis not only explores the 'what' of language, but also 'how' and 'why' experiences are told in certain ways, including the cultural resources individuals draw on and what is achieved through telling in particular ways. The construction of identity within narratives is also a performative social act involving not only the 'what' and 'how' of what is spoken, but also the question of to what purposes (Reissman, 2008). As part of attending to the symbolic aspects of identity, I noted how individuals actively constructed and performed their identities within narratives and interviews because this brought additional insights into individual agency (Maxwell and Aggleton, 2010) as well as how present identities relate to past ones (Reay, 1997). Thus, the narrative analyses I conducted attended to the what, how and why of the stories offered to me. The first practical step in the narrative analysis involved re-writing individual stories into biographical accounts so that their overall structure could be examined (Riessman, 2008). In the next step,

I undertook a thematic analysis of the data *within* the individual narratives, in contrast to the initial thematic analysis across the interviews in each data set, thereby keeping the accounts more intact than in traditional thematic analysis (Riessman, 2008). Within this process, I attended to the themes in the content of the narrative, including how individuals drew causal relationships between events (Taylor, 2006) and the historical and social contexts of the narratives (Riessman, 2008).

Discourse analysis was also part of the analytic approach for all three studies and aimed to explore the structuring effects of language within individual explanations of experiences and the subject positions available within these. The method of discourse analysis used here was most closely associated with the Foucauldian-informed approach of Parker (1992) and Burman and Parker (1993), which includes particular attention to the way language mirrors and reproduces power relations. While there is no one definitive approach to discourse analysis, Burman and Parker (1993) suggest that they share 'a concern with the ways language produces and constrains meaning, where meaning does not, or does not only, reside within the individual's head, and where social conditions give rise to the forms of talk available' (Burman and Parker, 1993: 3). Thus, 'meanings are multiple and shifting, rather than unitary and fixed' (Burman and Parker, 1993: 3). Because I pay significant attention to the effects of psychological theories in my research, I have employed discourse analytic approaches that were developed within critical psychology.

Turning to the specific steps undertaken in the discursive analysis of the interviews and qualitative survey text, I was guided by the criteria and associated steps for discourse analysis outlined by Parker (1992). I will not outline all of these in detail here, but instead describe some of the most pivotal steps in the process. As noted earlier, I categorised the data according to themes first: Parker (1992) suggests doing this later, after discourses have been initially identified, but I wanted to have a sense of the main themes across the data sets before I began identifying discourses. This was also helpful because I was dealing with three different data sets and it enabled me to see some thematic commonalities, such as the themes about the impact of abuse on sense of self. Once this process of thematic categorisation was complete, I attended to what objects and subjects were referred to in the data (Parker, 1992). This largely involved examining the way the objects of 'gendered violence and abuse' and 'mental health and illness' were constructed, followed by consideration of how the subjects, primarily 'abused women with mental health problems', were constructed. The approach specifically involved attention to how subjects were placed in a relation of power (Parker, 1992). For example, I show how humanist psychological discourses about lost sense of self and identity through abuse positioned women as having deficient, pathologised identities. Parker (1992) also suggests that a discourse refers to other discourses. This point deals with the issue of reflexivity, whereby 'the articulation of our reflections on discourse must require the use of discourses' (Parker, 1992: 13). Thus, in deconstructing humanist psychological discourses, I drew on a post-structural feminist discourse that is suspicious of essentialist notions of selfhood and their gendered effects, and thereby demonstrate the inherently gendered nature of these discourses. Parker (1992) also argues that 'analysis is facilitated by identifying contradictions between different ways of describing something', and that we need to understand the interrelationship between different discourses (Parker, 1992: 13). This necessitates setting contrasting discourses against each other, and looking at the different objects they constitute. This point is particularly pertinent to this study, in view of how central gender contradictions became in women's explanations of their experiences. Lastly, I attempt to provide a sense of how common particular discourses were within participants' accounts as part of establishing which might be considered dominant and which secondary.

I noted in the introduction to this chapter that navigating a path between the discursive and the material is no easy task. In the processes of data analysis described above, this necessitated attention to how narratives were constructed, the discourses being drawn on to explain understandings and experiences, the social contexts framing this, *and* women's lived experiences. However, while far from simple and straightforward – in fact at times quite messy – it was possible to distinguish to some extent between discourse and lived experience in women's talk. While I accept that all experience is mediated by language and therefore socially constructed, I could discern points in the data when women mobilised recognisable discourses to *explain* their lives, and other times when they spoke more 'from the heart' about their struggles and feelings. For example, women who had experienced domestic violence sometimes adopted psychological trauma discourses in order to construct a more social, non-pathologising understanding of their emotional distress. At other times they spoke with grief and anger about the losses domestic violence had wrought in their lives. While their talk about anger and grief was framed by contemporary discourses about individual rights and feminist discourses about gender equality, which made talking this way even possible, the women's descriptions of their grief, anger and isolation were not solely reducible to discourse because they included their lived, felt experience. This is not to suggest that some of what the women talked about represented 'truth' while other talk was merely discursive, but that visceral, bodily experiences emerged at times and these often spoke to the lived emotionality of gendered violence and abuse.

Another word about causation

It is important that I reiterate my comments on the issue of causation, given the focus of this research on gendered violence, abuse and mental health. In exploring women's experiences of mental health problems in contexts of gendered violence and abuse, I want to emphasise that I am not concerned with establishing a linear causative relationship between the two. It is widely agreed that the causes of mental health problems are multidimensional, involving sociocultural, psychological, familial and biological aspects, with no one factor explanatory on its own. At the same time, though, while I do not seek to 'prove' causation, many feminist researchers and scholars are prepared to assert that gendered violence and abuse cause mental health problems for women (for example, Humphreys and Thiara, 2003; Itzin *et al.*, 2010). While such claims are likely to be disputed by positivist scientists, medicine often overlooks the social causes and dimensions of health problems in favour of individual genetic ones (Willis, 1998). This reflects a bias towards biological reductionism and determinism based on assumptions that the 'real' causes of illness must lie within individual bodies because, otherwise, everyone would be 'sick'. This biological bias is also pertinent to multi-factorial models of the causes of ill-health, where individual, psychological and familial factors are often given much more weight than the socio-cultural dimensions (Krieger, 1994). Thus, narratives of causation are subject to interests and power relations, like all truth claims. It is important that, as feminists, we do not become too 'hung up' about causation but it is also important that we do not shy away from it. What I mean is that we ought not falsely seek to prove or claim causation through methods that are not designed to do so, but nor should we ignore the overwhelming evidence from positivist research that so firmly connects experiences of gendered violence with poor mental health and wellbeing for women. I now turn to the first of the three studies outlined above to consider how gender frames women's and men's experiences of childhood emotional abuse.

Note

1 The data on domestic violence and mental health was gathered as part of the following study: Franzway, S., Wendt, S., Moulding, N.T., Zufferey, C. and Chung, D.: 'Gendered violence and citizenship: the complex effects of intimate partner violence on mental health, housing and employment'. The study is funded by the Australian Research Council as a Discovery Project, No.: DP1130104437.

References

Althusser, L. (1971) *Lenin and Philosophy and Other Essays*. London: New Left Books.

Armstrong, L. (1994) *Rocking the Cradle of Sexual Politics: What Happened When Women Said Incest?* London: The Women's Press.

Braun, V. and Clarke, V. (2006) Using thematic analysis in psychology, *Qualitative Research in Psychology*, 3, pp. 77–101.

Broom, D.H. (1991) *Damned If We Do: Contradictions in Women's Health Care.* Sydney: Allen & Unwin.

Broverman, I.K., Vogel, S.R., Broverman, D.M., Clarkson, F.E. and Rosenkrantz, P.S. (1972) Sex-role stereotypes: a critical appraisal, *Journal of Social Issues*, 28, pp. 59–78.

Bryant, L. and Hoon, E. (2006) How can the intersections between gender, class, and sexuality be translated to an empirical agenda? *International Journal of Qualitative Methods*, 5(1), pp. 67–79.

Burman, E. and Parker, I. (1993) Introduction – discourse analysis: the turn to text. In E. Burman and I. Parker (eds), *Discourse Analytic Research: Readings and Repertoires of Texts in Action.* London: Routledge, pp. 1–13.

Burman, E., Alldred, P., Bewley, C., Goldberg, B., Heenan, C., Marks, D., Marshall, J., Taylor, K., Ullah, R. and Warner, S. (1996) *Challenging Women: Psychology's Exclusions, Feminist Possibilities*. Buckingham: Open University Press.

Butler, J. (1993) *Bodies That Matter: On the Discursive Limits of Sex*. New York: Routledge.

Chesler, P. (2005) *Women and Madness*. New York: Palgrave Macmillan.

Clough, P.T. and Halley, J. (2007) *The Affective Turn: Theorizing the Social*. Durham, NC: Duke University Press.

Crawford, J., Kippax, S., Onyx, J., Gault, U. and Benton, P. (1992). *Emotion and Gender: Constructing Meaning From Memory*. London: Sage Publications.

Faludi, S. (2006) *Backlash: The Undeclared War Against Women*. New York: Three Rivers Press.

Foucault, M. (1972) *The Archaeology of Knowledge*. London: Tavistock Publications Limited.

Foucault, M. (1977a) *Discipline and Punish: The Birth of the Prison*. London: Penguin Books.

Foucault, M. (1977b) Nietzsche, genealogy, history. In D.F. Bouchard (ed.), *Language, Counter-Memory, Practice: Selected Essays and Interviews*. New York: Cornell University Press, pp. 139–164.

Foucault, M. (1978) *The History of Sexuality Volume 1: An Introduction*. London: Penguin Books.

Foucault, M. (1980) *Power/Knowledge: Selected Interviews and Other Writings, 1972–1977*. Brighton: Harvester.

Foucault, M. (1982) The subject and power. In H. Dreyfus and P. Rabinow (eds), *Michel Foucault: Beyond Structuralism and Hermeneutics*. Chicago: University of Chicago Press, pp. 208–226.

Foucault, M. (1988) *The History of Sexuality Volume 3: The Care of the Self*. New York: Vintage Books.

Frank, A.W. (1995) *The Wounded Storyteller: Body, Illness and Ethics*. Chicago and London: University of Chicago Press.

Fraser, N. (2000) Rethinking recognition, *New Left Review*, 3, pp. 107–120.

Grbich, C. (1999) *Qualitative Research in Health: An Introduction*. St Leonards: Allen & Unwin.

Haaken, J. (2003) Traumatic revisions: remembering abuse and the politics of revision. In P. Reavey and S. Warner (eds), *New Feminist Stories of Child Sexual Abuse: Sexual Scripts and Dangerous Dialogues*. London: Routledge, pp. 131–147.

Henriques, J., Hollway, W., Urwin, C., Venn, C. and Walkerdine, V. (1984) *Changing the Subject: Psychology, Social Regulation and Subjectivity*. London: Methuen and Co. Ltd.

Herman, J.L. (1997) *Trauma and Recovery*. New York: Basic Books.

Humphreys, C. and Thiara, R. (2003) Mental health and domestic violence: 'I call it symptoms of abuse', *British Journal of Social Work*, 33(2), pp. 209–226.

Itzin, C., Taket, A. and Barter-Godfrey, S. (2010) *Domestic and Sexual Violence and Abuse: Tackling the Health and Mental Health Effects*. Abingdon: Routledge.

Jaggar, A.M. (1989) Love and knowledge: emotion in feminist epistemology. In A. Garry and M. Pearsall (eds), *Women, Knowledge and Reality: Explorations in Feminist Philosophy*. London: Unwin Hyman, pp. 129–155.

Kingdon, J. (1995) *Agendas, Alternatives, and Public Policies*, second edition. New York: HarperCollins.

Krieger, N. (1994) Epidemiology and the web of causation: has anyone seen the spider? *Social Science and Medicine*, 39(7), pp. 887–993.

Lamb, S. (1999) Constructing the victim: popular images and lasting labels. In S. Lamb (ed.), *New Versions of Victims: Feminist Struggle with the Concept*. New York and London: New York University Press, pp. 108–138.

Lloyd, G. (1989). The man of reason. In A. Garry and M. Pearsall (eds), *Women, Knowledge and Reality: Explorations in Feminist Philosophy*. London: Unwin Hyman, pp. 111–128.

McNay, L. (1992) *Foucault and Feminism: Power, Gender and the Self*. Oxford: Polity Press.

McNay, L. (2004) Situated intersubjectivity. In B. Marshall and A. Witz (eds), *Engendering the Social: Feminist Encounters with Sociological Theory*. Maidenhead: Open University Press, pp. 171–186.

McNay, L. (2008) *Against Recognition*. Cambridge: Polity Press.

Malson, H. (1998) *The Thin Woman: Feminism, Post-Structuralism and the Social Psychology of Anorexia Nervosa*. London: Routledge.

Maxwell, C. and Aggleton, P. (2010) Agency in action: young women and their sexual relationships in a private school, *Gender and Education*, 22(3), pp. 327–343.

Mishler, E.G. (1997) The interactional construction of narratives in medical and life-history interviews. In B.L. Gunnarsson, P. Linell and B. Norbert (eds), *The Construction of Professional Discourse*. London and New York: Longman, pp. 223–244.

Moulding, N.T. (2003) Constructing the self in mental health practice: identity, individualism and the feminisation of deficiency, *Feminist Review*, 75, pp. 57–74.

Moulding, N.T. (2006) Disciplining the feminine: the reproduction of gender contradictions in the mental health care of women with eating disorders, *Social Science & Medicine*, 62(4), pp. 793–804.

Oakley, A. (1981) Interviewing women: a contradiction in terms. In H. Roberts (ed.), *Doing Feminist Research*. London: Routledge and Kegan Paul, pp. 31–61.

O'Dell, L. (2003) The 'harm' story in child sexual abuse: contested understandings, disputed knowledges. In P. Reavey and S. Warner (eds), *New Feminist Stories of Child Sexual Abuse: Sexual Scripts and Dangerous Dialogues*. London: Routledge, pp. 131–147.

Parker, I. (1992) *Discourse Dynamics: Critical Analysis for Social and Individual Psychology*. London: Routledge.

Parker, I., Georgaca, E., Harper, D., McLaughlin, T. and Stowell-Smith, M. (1995) *Deconstructing Psychopathology*. London: Sage Publications.

Probyn, E. (1993) *Sexing the Self: Gendered Positions in Cultural Studies*. London: Routledge.

Reavey, P. and Warner, S. (2003) Introduction. In P. Reavey and S. Warner (eds), *New Feminist Stories of Child Sexual Abuse: Sexual Scripts and Dangerous Dialogues*. London: Routledge, pp. 1–12.

Reay, D. (1997) Feminist theory, habitus, and social class: disrupting notions of classlessness, *Women's Studies International Forum*, 20(2), pp. 225–233.

Riessman, C.K. (2008) *Narrative Methods for the Human Sciences*. Thousand Oaks: Sage.

Sarantakos, S. (2012) *Social Research*, fourth edition. South Yarra: Macmillan Education Australia Pty Ltd.

Sawicki, J. (1991) *Disciplining Foucault: Feminism, Power and the Body*. New York: Routledge.

Stanley, L. and Wise, S. (1990) Method, methodology and epistemology in feminist research processes. In L. Stanley (ed.), *Feminist Praxis: Research, Theory and Epistemology in Feminist Sociology*. London: Routledge, pp. 20–60.

Taylor, S. (2006) Narrative as construction and discursive resource, *Narrative Inquiry*, 16(1), pp. 94–102.

Taylor, S. and Littleton, K. (2006) Biographies in talk: a narrative-discursive approach, *Qualitative Sociology Review*, 11(1), pp. 22–38.

Ussher, J. (1991) *Women's Madness: Misogyny or Mental Illness?* Harlow: Prentice Hall.

Ussher, J. (2010) Are we medicalizing women's misery: a critical review of women's higher rates of reported depression, *Feminism and Psychology*, 20(9), pp. 9–35.

Walby, S. (1990) *Theorizing Patriarchy*. Cambridge, MA: Blackwell Publishers.

Walby, S. (2006) Patriarchy. In J. Scott (ed.), *Sociology: Key Concepts*. London: Routledge, pp. 121–123.

Walby, S., Towers, J. and Francis, B. (2014) Mainstreaming domestic and gender-based violence into sociology and the criminology of violence, *The Sociological Review*, 62(S2), pp. 187–214.

Warner, S. (2009) *Understanding the Effects of Child Sexual Abuse: Feminist Revolutions in Theory, Research and Practice*. London: Routledge.

Weedon, C. (1987) *Feminist Practice and Poststructuralist Theory*. Oxford: Basil Blackwell.

Wendt, S. and Zannettino, L. (2015) *Domestic Violence in Diverse Contexts: A Re-Examination of Gender*. London: Routledge.

Williams, R. (1977) *Marxism and Literature*. Oxford: Oxford University Press.

Willis, E. (1998) Public health, private genes: the social context of genetic biotechnologies, *Critical Public Health*, 8(2), pp. 131–139.

Wirth-Cauchon, J. (2001) *Borderline Personality Disorder: Symptoms and Stories*. Piscataway: Rutgers University Press.

World Health Organization (WHO) (2013) *Global and Regional Estimates of Violence against Women: Prevalence and Health Effects of Intimate Partner Violence and Non-Partner Sexual Violence*. Geneva: WHO. Available at: www.who.int/reproductive-health/publications/violence/9789241564625/en/, accessed 22 April 2015.

4 Childhood emotional abuse

Engendering selves, engendering bodies

Childhood emotional abuse has received much less attention than other forms of interpersonal abuse, but it is now increasingly focused on by researchers and clinicians as awareness of child sexual abuse has grown over the past three decades. While childhood emotional abuse is arguably the most difficult to define, it cannot be understood as a single, universal phenomenon because it varies enormously, and is interpreted and experienced differently by individuals (Pelcovitz *et al.*, 1994). More specifically, like all forms of interpersonal abuse, childhood emotional abuse is framed by specific social relations of gender, race and class (May-Chahal, 2006). However, most of the research into childhood emotional abuse and mental health sits within psychology and takes a gender-neutral, positivist approach that detaches abuse from the meaning individuals themselves attribute to it and the social context within which it takes place. Hence, few studies have specifically considered the gender dimensions and dynamics of childhood emotional abuse, nor those associated with race and class: the gendered and other social dimensions of this phenomenon therefore remain little understood. Other than the research I have undertaken and draw on in this chapter, then, no other feminist research has been conducted in this area to date. In undertaking this research, though, my purpose was not to 'prove' the existence or otherwise of gender differences in experiences of childhood emotional abuse. Rather, what I am concerned with is elaborating the discourses framing women's and men's narratives and experiences of childhood emotional abuse, the related social practices and the relationship of these discourses and practices to wider gender and other social inequalities.

Psycho-medical theorisations

As noted in Chapter 2, a widely accepted definition suggests that it involves 'a verbal assault on a child's sense of worth and wellbeing, or any humiliating, demeaning or threatening behaviour directed toward a child by an older person' (Bernstein and Fink, 1998: 2). Doyle (2001) refers to a long-standing definition from Hart *et al.* (1983) of childhood emotional abuse as involving acts of omission and commission by parents that, in the light of community standards and professional perspectives, are understood to be psychologically damaging.

According to Glaser (2002), emotional abuse involves a repeated pattern of damaging interactions of commission and omission that can convey a sense of worthlessness, being unloved, flawed, unwanted or in danger or only of value in meeting someone else's needs, that is, regard is only conditional. Boulton and Hindle (2000) also argue that emotional abuse is an inherent part of all types of interpersonal abuse. As noted in Chapter 2, class and race are also specifically relevant to childhood emotional abuse, as they are to all abuse, because poorer groups experience much more surveillance of their child-rearing practices. Moreover, vastly divergent phenomena can be captured within the constructs of physical and emotional abuse so that practices considered abusive in one context might be understood as forms of discipline in another (May-Chahal, 2006).

Estimations of the prevalence of childhood emotional abuse were outlined in Chapter 2 along with research into the connections between this form of abuse and poor mental health. In this chapter, I critically examine the way these connections are theorised in the psycho-medical literature. While the links between childhood emotional abuse and mental health problems have been well-established, many psychological studies are concerned with elucidating specific cognitive processes as 'mediators' of the relationship between abuse and mental illness. The purpose of this type of research is to try and explain the mechanisms through which abuse leads to mental health problems, but also why some individuals go on to develop mental health problems and others do not. For example, O'Dougherty Wright *et al.* (2009) focus on the idea that childhood emotional abuse and later distress is 'mediated' by 'maladaptive schemas' such as vulnerability to harm, self-sacrifice and shame. Maciejewski and Mazure (2006) examine 'fear of criticism and rejection' and its role in mediation between childhood emotional abuse and depression. Not dissimilarly, Sachs-Ericsson *et al.* (2010) examine self-criticism as 'mediating' the relationship between parental verbal abuse and what they call 'internalising disorders' of anxiety and depression. Other studies have looked at 'restrained adult style of emotional expression' (Krause *et al.*, 2003). These types of studies understand cognitive and emotional 'styles' or 'patterns' as relatively fixed and unchanging in the individual, and detach individual subjectivity from its social context. They also seek to distinguish supposedly psychopathological responses to abuse from 'normal' psychological functioning. Some of these researchers also draw on other more general psychological theories to explain how emotional abuse results in mental health problems, with attachment theory currently the most popular. Attachment theory focuses on the idea that insecure attachment with a primary caregiver, who is almost always assumed to be the mother, causes psychological problems in children through to adulthood (Bowlby, 1988). For example, Coates (2010) looks at neurobiology and social contexts of abuse but draws on attachment theory as the main explanation for why abuse can lead to mental health problems. O'Dougherty Wright *et al.* (2009) also centre attachment theory as the main explanation for how 'maladaptive schemas' result in psychopathology following abuse. The obvious weakness in this approach is that a substantial proportion of childhood emotional abuse is perpetrated by fathers, who are usually not the primary caregivers of children. Other researchers focus on the idea of emotional abuse as causing low self-esteem (for example, Sachs-Ericsson *et al.*, 2010). Kennedy *et al.* (2007) suggest that childhood emotional abuse is particularly linked to low self-esteem and poor mental health because it can be more easily construed as 'a personal attack on the self' than other types of child abuse (p. 19). Emotional abuse also directly supplies the child with a negative sense of themselves, such as 'I am worthless' (Sachs-Ericsson *et al.*, 2010: 492) and can therefore be understood as an attack on another's integrity (Krause *et al.*, 2003). However, even low self-esteem is explained in the language of pathology in much of this research, for example, as so-called deficits in self-concept (Rorty and Yager, 1996) or as indicative of 'psychopathology' (Mullen *et al.*, 1996).

In addition to the examination of supposedly fixed psychological constructs and patterns in individuals, some of the psychological research also considers the emotional impact of abuse. This aspect of the psychological research can be somewhat less pathologising and more insightful than that concerned with establishing psychopathological constructs and patterns. A number of studies have shown that childhood emotional abuse is associated with powerful and often enduring feelings of shame, worthlessness, humiliation and anger (Harper and Arias, 2004; Krause *et al.*, 2003; O'Dougherty Wright *et al.*, 2009). O'Dougherty Wright *et al.* (2009) suggest that shame and sense of defectiveness from emotional abuse is based on the idea that the core self has not lived up to expectations. Moreover, shaming in emotional abuse takes place in an ongoing relationship rather than simply within specific events, which may in part explain its long-term, injurious effects (O'Dougherty Wright *et al.*, 2009).

Harper and Arias (2004) specifically explored shame and how it might explain the relation between childhood emotional abuse and adult anger and depression. They cite research which shows that childhood psychological abuse is positively correlated with proneness to shame while physical abuse is not (Hoglund and Nicholas, 1995, cited in Harper and Arias, 2004). The authors point out that shame is commonly understood as an emotion that is primarily about defeat and submission but they argue that there is also overt and bypassed shame (Lewis, 1971, cited in Harper and Arias, 2004). Overt shame involves acknowledgement and an acute feeling of utter humiliation and failure, as in wanting to 'die of shame', as well as self-blame for events so that they are seen as stemming from the individual's bad self (Harper and Arias, 2004). Overt shame is thought to result in sadness and depression while bypassed shame is seen to be associated with avoidance and denial of shame, and is theorised as leading to the externalisation of anger and hostility (Harper and Arias, 2004). Harper and Arias (2004) measured childhood emotional abuse and shame in 373 college students in the United States, and they reported that women experience higher levels of shame in response to childhood emotional abuse than men. Moreover, for women, more shame equalled more negative reactions to abuse and higher levels of 'internalised' responses such as depression. Men, they argue, experienced increased anger in response to shame from childhood emotional abuse, which allows them to bypass or avoid feelings of shame and pain and therefore regain a sense of control over their negative feelings about themselves (Harper and Arias, 2004). While this research throws some light on internalisation versus externalisation of feelings according to gender and its links to shame, the authors give little attention to how or why these differences might occur other than to suggest that 'women may be more likely to experience overt shame as a result of a tendency toward rumination and self-focus' (Harper and Arias, 2004: 373). In not elaborating further, they perhaps inadvertently leave the reader to draw the conclusion that these observed differences must be the work of biological sex differences. Interestingly, the authors did not predict any gender differences in relation to shame from childhood emotional abuse, having framed their study in entirely gender-neutral terms, and they come across as quite surprised by their findings.

Gender neutral or gender blind?

The above-mentioned study by Harper and Arias (2004) addressed gender by default because it arose so strongly in the findings but, as pointed out, their study was framed from the outset in gender-neutral terms, as is the case with almost all of the psychological research into childhood emotional abuse. As noted in Chapter 2, the gender-neutral approach is reinforced by the fact that all the pre-determined scales used to measure emotional abuse fail to actually ask what was said to the individual, by who or in what context, opting to group emotionally abusive practices by type instead. In addition to failing to attend to the content of abuse, O'Dougherty Wright et al. (2009) treat gender as a 'predictor variable' based on the fact that another study (that by Harper and Arias, 2004) had found powerful gender differences in shame responses to childhood emotional abuse. Thus, rather than exploring gender further, they seem to treat it as a confounding variable and to some extent write it out of analysis. Intriguingly, a number of other studies specifically explore the effects of childhood emotional abuse in women, but fail to explain why they have chosen to look at women in particular (for example, Mullen et al., 1996). Again, this failure to address gender directly perhaps inadvertently implies that women are simply biologically prone to more negative responses to abuse or there is an unspoken assumption of women as 'natural victims'.

Downs and colleagues have undertaken two of the only psychological studies that consider the gendered dimensions of childhood emotional abuse (Downs and Miller, 1998; Downs and Rindels, 2004). In the first study, Downs and Miller (1998) distinguished between abuse perpetrated by mothers and fathers, and the effects on daughters and sons, and set out to compare the impact of abuse along these lines. As noted earlier, they found that fathers' abuse predicted mental health problems in daughters but not in sons, while mothers' abuse did not predict problems in either daughters or sons. In previous research, these authors had also found that women's alcoholism is related to fathers' violence but not mothers'. They suggest that fathers' violence might be more physically and psychologically threatening to girls because of men's greater power in the family and the greater physical impact of his violence against which girls are less able to defend themselves (Downs and Miller, 1998). To reinforce their argument, they point to

Pelcovitz *et al.*'s (1994) finding that items of abuse defined objectively by researchers are of less concern to young people than the experiences they themselves define as abusive. Downs and Miller (1998) also suggest that girls might receive more support from mothers, too, which might counter some of the abuse perpetrated by them, pointing to another study that found that girls found mothers' loving behaviours more supportive than boys did. This same study is reported as finding that girls also rate a father's emotional and physical abuse as more abusive than boys do. Downs and Rindels (2004) suggest that abusive fathers in particular can have a long-term negative impact on girls that lasts well into adulthood. Further to this, they found that having an absent father is better for girls than having a father who is present but abusive. Again, the authors seemed surprised by these findings, appearing not to have predicted that abusive fathers might have such a negative impact on girls. Perhaps this reflects how established are negative discourses about female-headed single parent families in the United States such that any father is assumed to be better than none at all.

While the studies conducted by Downs and colleagues are important because they draw attention to the differential impact of abuse on women and men according to who perpetrates the abuse, like other psychological research, the authors never consider the specific content or context of the abuse itself because they, too, use scales that group different types of abusive practices together. Verbal denigration can involve completely different social meanings depending on what is said, how it is said and by whom. For example, being called a 'slut' is qualitatively different to being called 'lazy'. A boy is highly unlikely to be called a 'slut', whereas a girl is quite highly likely to encounter this insult. But even if a boy were called a 'slut', the meaning and impact would be quite different because it is a fundamentally *gendered* insult that is usually reserved for women and girls, and only has real meaning in this context. Downs and colleagues also fail to consider that what mothers might say and do as part of abuse might also be quite qualitatively different to what fathers might say and do. Moreover, also in common with all of the psychological research in this area, the wider social context of gender inequalities is entirely absent from the picture.

In addition to the body of quantitative psychological research into childhood emotional abuse, two qualitative studies have been undertaken. Doyle (2001) interviewed 14 women and men about their experiences of childhood emotional abuse with a focus on what helped them overcome the impact of abuse in their lives. Based on her own experience of undertaking both quantitative and qualitative research in this area, Doyle (2001) argues that quantitative methods are inadequate in this area and that qualitative research can give us a much more comprehensive picture. She found that other family members were identified as most important to coping, particularly aunts, however, the non-offending parent was not among these. While this research was able to provide a much more nuanced account of the diversity of individual experience and gave voice to individuals who had been abused, it did not attend to the gendered, raced or classed dimensions of abuse but offered a more individual, phenomenological perspective. Thomas and Hall (2008) studied 44 women's narratives of recovery after child abuse, including emotional abuse. They identified four types of redemption narratives: redemption through counselling or psychotherapy, redemption through the experience of a loving relationship, self-redemption and redemption by god. They draw attention to the 'hard work' of what they call 'thriving' after childhood abuse. The identification of redemption narratives is useful in showing the different social and cultural resources women draw on to overcome the effects of abuse, and this study also provides very detailed insights into the different ways women managed their lives after abuse. However, the authors never explain why they have specifically focused on women and nor do they attend at all to the ways gender might frame women's experiences. For example, they point out that many of the abused women went on to have 'disastrous marriages' and they also identify how important raising healthy children was to overcoming abuse, but they do not consider how gender might frame these aspects of the narratives.

Researching the gendered dimensions of childhood emotional abuse

As was pointed out in Chapter 2, while feminist researchers have given much attention to child sexual abuse, as yet there have been no feminist studies of childhood emotional abuse. As such, the empirical research reported here is the first attempt to examine the phenomenon of childhood emotional abuse from a feminist perspective. Also as argued in Chapter 2, while both mothers and fathers are involved in childhood emotional abuse, examination of its gendered dimensions extends beyond counts of the gender of perpetrators and victims to explore how gender discourses and power relations frame practices of emotional abuse. In line with the theoretical and methodological approach of all the primary research in this book, the study was framed by McNay's (2004) concept of situated intersubjectivity in seeking to attend to both the discursive or symbolic aspects of individual explanations of childhood emotional abuse and to the material, lived realities of these experiences and their implications for mental health and wellbeing. I draw here on data from two studies – the study of childhood emotional abuse and the study into experiences of gendered abuse in women who have developed eating disorders. I have drawn on both studies because five of the women in the eating disorder study placed an emphasis on childhood emotional abuse in their explanations of their experiences. Together, these studies comprise a sample of 17 individuals with backgrounds of childhood emotional abuse, 13 women and four men, with one of the women (Louise) contributing interviews for both studies. Both women and men were invited into the studies, however, no men took part in the eating disorder study and only a small number participated in the emotional abuse study. Eight of the participants were under 25 years of age, two were aged between 25 and 40 years, and seven were aged between 40 and 55 years. The sample was reasonably diverse in terms of class background, with eight participants reporting working-class or socially disadvantaged backgrounds, eight reporting middle-class backgrounds and one reporting an upper-class background. However, most of the participants were undertaking tertiary studies at the time of the interviews because some recruitment was on campus, mainly in the human service professions, with one woman an administrative worker and another a community worker. Cultural backgrounds included some diversity, with most participants Anglo-Celtic and one reporting an Indigenous Australian background. In addition to this, there was one participant each from the following cultural backgrounds: South-east Asian, Middle-Eastern, Eastern European and Southern European. Other than the participant from the Middle East who had migrated with her family within the last 15 years, all were second- or third-generation Australian. Seven participants described families where one or both parents had a mental illness (six mothers and one father), one father was described as having had a significant drinking problem and five participants described highly conflictual relationships between the parents, although none of these were named as domestic violence. Two of the mothers who were reported as having serious mental illnesses were also thought to have been sexually abused by their fathers as children. Eight of the participants, seven women and one man, disclosed sexual abuse in addition to emotional abuse while five reported physical abuse.

In three cases, participants described both their father and mother as emotionally abusive; in six cases fathers were described as the abusers; and in five cases mothers were described as abusive. One man described his older sister as sexually and emotionally abusive, while two women reported physical and emotional abuse from older brothers and another two reported sexual abuse from older brothers. One woman also described her grandfather as perpetrating sexual abuse in addition to emotional abuse from both her parents. While female participants reported abuse by fathers, mothers, brothers and grandfathers, male participants reported parental abuse only from fathers, in addition to the one male who reported abuse from his older sister. Women therefore reported a wider range of abuse from a broader cross-section of relatives than men. Two participants, one woman and one man, also reported bullying from peers, and in the case of the male participant, this was race-related.

Participants were asked to describe the emotional abuse they had experienced, including what was said, by whom and in what context. They were also asked to explain how they understood the relationship between their experiences of abuse and their mental health and wellbeing. The following analysis focuses primarily on the gendered dimensions of childhood emotional abuse. However, there were many aspects of emotional abuse that were reported by both women and men. First, there was some agreement about what participants saw as constituting emotional abuse. This included the verbal abuse and denigration of children; the misuse of power by belittling children to make them feel 'less' than the adult; preventing children from having and expressing emotions; scapegoating children; and showing no empathy towards children. Many participants also said that they did not recognise that their families were abusive until they visited their friends' homes as children or adolescents. Thus, high levels of emotional abuse and conflict were 'normal' to them as children and only became remarkable when they realised that not all families behaved like this. Second, many participants suggested that their parents were themselves emotionally, physically or sexually abused in childhood, and there was a significant related discourse about the re-enactment of abuse in families (see Boulton and Hindle, 2000, for discussion of this). Third, many of these parents, as well as other abusive parents discussed by the participants, were also described as struggling with significant mental illnesses, which were presented as driving the abuse to some extent. Without disputing the reality of mental illness among the participants' parents, a significant 'abuser-as-ill' discourse continues to prevail in this area and was arguably present in the participants' narratives (Bell, 2011). The participants also identified experiencing a host of mental health problems which they traced to their experiences of emotional abuse including anxiety, particularly PTSD and panic; depression; bipolar disorder; dissociative identity disorder in one of the women who was also severely sexually abused; eating disorders, but only in the women; and anti-social personality disorder, or sociopathic personality, in the one man who also reported sexual abuse. In line with the research evidence about the effects of abuse on mental health (Messman-Moore and Garrigus, 2007), the most serious mental health problems of severe PTSD, dissociative identity disorder, severe eating disorders and sociopathic personality all involved both emotional abuse and extensive intra-familial sexual abuse that was usually denied within the family.

Femininities and masculinities in narratives of childhood emotional abuse

In addition to the more general experiences of childhood emotional abuse outlined above, participants also described abuse focused on areas stereotypically associated with either femininity or masculinity. The nature of the interview questions enabled this to emerge because I purposely asked participants to tell me what was said, how, by whom and in what context. Hence, the women described being emotionally abused about their appearance, weight and sexualities; the use of emotional abuse to force them into unwanted domestic and caring duties; and they described being given 'mixed messages' about who they were or what they were supposed to achieve in life. The men described abuse for being insufficiently 'manly'; being pushed to achieve in sports; or abuse focused on achievement in work or in their studies. Significant aspects of their narratives were therefore focused around areas of traditional masculine achievement. Thus, femininities and masculinities were central to these aspects of the narratives, with the discourses and practices of femininity in the women's narratives demonstrating significant levels of contradiction, while those associated with masculinities in the men's accounts were more hegemonic.

R.W. Connell (2005) has explored gender and masculinities in some depth. She talks about 'doing gender', arguing that gender is interactional and 'a way in which social practice is ordered' so that 'when we speak of masculinity and femininity we are naming configurations of gender practice' (pp. 71–72). Further to this, while she argues that femininities and masculinities involve internal contradiction and disruption, and are not fixed in time and place, at any given time there is nonetheless a 'hegemonic masculinity' (Connell, 2005). She borrows from Antonio Gramsci's concept of hegemony as 'the cultural dynamic by which a group claims and sustains a leading position in social life' (Connell, 2005: 77). In applying hegemony to masculinities, R.W. Connell (2005) argues that hegemonic masculinity is 'the configuration of gender practice which embodies the currently accepted answer to the problem of the legitimacy of patriarchy, which guarantees (or is taken to guarantee) the dominant position of men and the subordination of women' (p. 77). In her analysis of contemporary Australian masculinities, Connell (2005) reveals a diversity of masculinities that vary according to class, race, education and other categories of social difference. However, she identifies hegemonic masculinity, in particular, as establishing its power through the idea that it embodies the 'power of reason', as opposed to 'irrational', feminised emotion. The following analysis will show how the men drew on hegemonic masculinities that specifically centred the control of emotion in their narratives of childhood emotional abuse, and how this enabled them to use power and control in ways that brought a level of personal and social benefit. There was no counterpart to this for the women and, instead, highly contradictory femininity discourses and practices not uncommonly left them with ongoing feelings of self-doubt, responsibility and guilt, and related struggles with mental health. This is not to suggest that the men did not suffer, because they did, but that hegemonic masculinities also proffered a range of advantages in managing abuse that were simply unavailable to the women. Nor does this mean that the men only engaged with one single hegemonic masculinity in their day-to-day lives. Rather, in the specific activity of narrating childhood emotional abuse, hegemonic masculinities were central and beneficial to the men in a number of ways, but they also brought certain disadvantages, too.

Because the women's accounts involved many more contradictory discourses and experiences and the men's tended to congregate around more singular themes that built on each other, there is a different flavour to the two sections of the analysis. Thus, the women's stories are dealt with more thematically across the data while the men's enabled more of a narrative analysis in addition to analysis of key themes. In essence, what this shows is that childhood emotional abuse can be a powerful tool of engendering that risks entrenching gender differences along relatively binary lines, but I also show later in Chapter 8 how the participants, particularly the women, resisted or modified these binaries in their attempts to find other ways of being.

Women and childhood emotional abuse: controlling the feminine

In addition to abuse focused on feminised areas of responsibility and activity, two women first mentioned their more general observation that the emotional abuse they experienced was specifically concerned with placing controls on, and limitations around, their behaviour. Melissa specifically observed that the emotional abuse she experienced seemed mostly concerned with exacting her obedience to parental demands:

[My brother] got yelled at a lot, like now that I look back at it – I didn't realise at the time – but [he] got yelled at a lot for things he was meant to be responsible for, he was meant to be a man, he was meant to be responsible, and so he got yelled at for all those kinds of things. Whereas I got yelled at for not obeying, and not doing what I was told.

(Melissa)

Thus, Melissa described her brother being pressured to 'step up' to masculine responsibilities while she was chastised for not doing what she was told. Not dissimilarly, Rose said that her parents 'want to control me' and that her brother has been exempted from this:

He's a boy. In my family males are preferred … he doesn't have to clean, it's okay he's allowed to swear, little things like that.… She's more getting upset at him because he didn't kiss his mum for mother's day, something like that, so.… He's favoured.

(Rose)

Thus, emotional abuse was described as controlling, repressive and concerned with the enforcement of feminine responsibilities and behaviours, while brothers were exempted or sometimes seemed 'preferred' and allowed more latitude in their general behaviour. A number of women believed that their brothers were preferred over them and thereby protected to some extent from emotional abuse, particularly maternal emotional abuse.

Surveillance and control of female bodies

Some women described abuse that was specifically focused on their appearance, weight and sexualities, areas particularly associated with the feminine and the female body. Melissa said that she was called 'fat' by both her parents as part of emotional abuse, and that this 'shattered my self-confidence':

At the time, as well, it has definitely followed through into my adult years, it really shattered my self-confidence, because my dad would tell me I'm fat or.… I very much resented him for because he never looked after his own body weight – neither of my parents have and they are quite unhealthy themselves, so the fact that they would comment that 'Why do you eat so much, you look so fat'. It was like … ironic.

(Melissa)

Rose not dissimilarly described being called 'the fatty of the family':

I've always been the fatty of the family … I've always been the fatty … my brother has always called me [fatty] and my mum and dad laughed, he was only about three or four when he said it but it's been an ongoing thing because they laugh at it ... they've said the term but Carlo [my brother did it] in front of extended family members, very embarrassing yeah ... and kind of during puberty yeah so thunder thighs a couple of times at school, things like that with other people.... And my mum made me wear a girdle once when I was eight or nine ... and the dress was quite not tight but the fabric you could see all my lumps and bumps so she made me wear girdles when we went out.

(Rose)

Rose's account captures not only abuse from her immediate family about her weight but also public humiliation and shaming in the wider extended family. She went on to say that, as a result, 'I've definitely been more self-conscious'. Rebecca, who went on to experience anorexia followed by bulimia, described being called fat by her older brother, who had also sexually abused her, while Georgia described her father calling her fat once she reached puberty. Rose later drew attention to the 'no win' of body control for women when she talked about how getting fit by going to the gym also drew further emotional abuse about her body and appearance:

I can't win at all in my house so I've got a protein shake that ... after I go the gym I have it and it's so my muscles don't hurt the next day. It's not because I want to be a body builder.... And [my mother will] go 'what the hell is that for?' ... 'what are you, a man?' ... and 'what's with your hair, why is your makeup like that?'.

(Rose)

In this account, Rose is accused of turning herself 'into a man', but she also mentioned criticism about other aspects of her appearance such as her hair and make-up. This captures the sheer breadth and intrusiveness of the day-to-day body surveillance to which women are subjected and how this can be mobilised in childhood emotional abuse. It also captures the contradictions inherent to feminine body ideals because Rose is criticised for 'feminine flabbiness' but also for 'masculine muscle'. Of course the real point is that she is supposed to be thin and the abuse Rose described is therefore framed by her failure to comply with this contemporary feminine ideal.

A number of women also described emotionally abusive practices focused on their sexualities. Melissa's family are part of an evangelical Christian sect with extremist views about female modesty and highly patriarchal gender relations, with women in servile positions to the men. She described her parents' efforts to enforce modesty on her as repressive and abusive:

There was a lot more pressure on me physically about how I appeared.... And ... really one of the bigger things was that women according my dad and my mum ... they both believed at the time that women had to wear long skirts ... my mother gave me such a lecture when I went to church and I was wearing a cross between a dress and a shirt, and leggings, and – 'They're pants [.] and you're not allowed to wear pants, you have to wear skirts', and … I was getting in trouble for leggings, and … you know if I wore a low-cut top my dad would tell me I looked like a slut.

(Melissa)

Melissa mentioned being called a 'slut' by her father for wearing certain clothing, which draws on long-standing and dualistic historical discourses about women as either virgins or whores (MacSween, 1993). Melissa also described feelings of guilt about her bisexuality because she was subjected to very conservative Christian views about sex and sexuality, saying 'I've only been able to accept that about myself this year, because before, I was so convinced that I was just a sinful person and I was evil for feeling this way about girls'. She went on to describe struggling with significant anxiety and panic disorder as a young adult. Rebecca talked about being told that sex was 'dirty' and that her developing body was 'disgusting' as part of emotional abuse:

I always got messages that [sex] was dirty. My mum would say, 'now look, no playing around with guys before you get married, because you know it's dirty, you know, you just don't do that'. And my father would come in if I was, let's say I was 12, and my brother was 10, and we were getting ready for school and we were in front of the heater, and I had my underpants and my singlet on, and he'd say, 'get to your room, that's disgusting, like this in front of your brother'. And I said, 'oh, ok', you know what I mean?

(Rebecca)

Rebecca mentioned becoming increasingly ashamed and frightened of sex during puberty because of these negative messages about sex and female sexuality. Rose talked at some length about having her sexuality monitored and controlled. Rose is from a middle-class Italian background, and her parents were described as holding strong views about sex before marriage. Her mother was also portrayed as extremely concerned with family honour and how the family is seen in the community. Thus, in spite of the fact that Rose is an adult and well beyond the age of consent, she is not permitted to have a sexual relationship with her boyfriend. She said:

There's conflict between me and my Mum because I'd want to stay at my partner's house and that's a no-no so I'm not allowed to kind of, yeah, do anything. I'd love to move out of home but I don't think they would allow me to or support me doing that.

(Rose)

Rose also mentioned restrictions on her general independence, not just her sexuality, with the two tied together to some extent. Rose went on to describe other intrusive methods of surveillance used to monitor whether she is being sexual:

[My mother has] been quite like if she sees that I have tampons in my room or something and if I stay not stay at my boyfriend's house but I'm there until midnight, for example, she won't message me but if she doesn't know that I have my period or I don't have my period she will message me, 'Where are you? Get the [fuck] home. Where are you? It's late' ... so silly things like that. I've had to lie to her about being on the contraceptive pill.

(Rose)

This surveillance of private bodily processes was depicted as highly intrusive and shaming, and as forcing Rose to lie about her sexual life. Lastly, Aisha described emotional abuse by her father where he blamed her for a rape perpetrated by their next-door neighbour when she was 16 years old. She said:

In my culture it's, I don't know, they just, it's always your fault. I mean, they say, 'well you might have wanted it'. Because the problem was I was 16, I wasn't just like a five year old or someone who had no idea what's going on, and so I could have run, but I didn't. Or I could have screamed, but I didn't. So, that was the problem. So, my parents were quite mad at me for some time.

(Aisha)

Aisha drew on a number of victim-blaming discourses and practices to explain her father's reaction to the rape and while she links these specifically to her Middle-Eastern culture, similar discourses persist in Western cultures, if less overtly than in the past (Gavey, 2005; Gavey and Schmidt, 2011). First, the suggestion that she would be seen to have 'wanted it' is based on the idea that the 'dangerous, lurking' nature of female sexuality provokes rape, but also that women secretly want to be raped (Gavey, 2005: 19). Second, the assumption that a rape occurs because of insufficient resistance locates total responsibility on the woman to prevent unwanted sex: thus, in a quite stunning example of circular logic, if a rape takes place, the woman must really have wanted it (Gavey, 2005). Aisha went on to describe being grounded by her father for months to prevent contact with other men, and developing problems with anxiety, insomnia and a night-time binge-eating disorder when she later became estranged from her family, although she nonetheless continued to provide care for her mentally ill mother.

The imposition of domestic and caring duties

As noted, some women described abuse focused on cooking, cleaning and caring for children and other relatives. Catherine and Rose talked about verbal abuse about being 'messy', usually from mothers and focused on co-opting them into cleaning chores. Rose went on to describe emotional manipulation about pressure to undertake other household chores, too, such as cooking and shopping rather than doing her studies:

[My mother will] be saying how she had to go to the shops all day.... I had to do all of this for all of you and you come home and just sit down on your computers and you don't help me cook and we're like 'we're doing home-work mum'.

Q: And is this to your brother too?
A: No, she'll say all of you but he won't be listening, he'll be in there so she's really directing it at me ... [she yells] so it's very stressful.

(Rose)

Mothers tend to carry most if not all of the burden of cooking and cleaning in the family, and Rose's mother is depicted here as using guilt and inferences of self-ishness to recruit her into sharing this gendered burden. Also concerned with domestic duties, some women described abuse focused on forcing them to care for younger siblings or for the abusive parent themselves. Melissa told how she was made to care for her two disabled younger sisters while her parents went away for the weekend:

[My father] wanted me to stay home and look after the girls, but the thing is [both are disabled] ... and I was upset about it and I said 'I can't do it on my own' and he got really angry at me and he got right up close and started, like, stroking my cheek and going 'Oh, poor baby', like 'You're such a princess, and we always have to look after you, and you're such a pain', and things like that.... And I think that's the first time I ever swore at my dad, I turned around and I said 'Well, you think you're king shit', and he – I was scared he was going to slap me – he didn't, but my mum made me get down on my knees and beg him for forgiveness.... They made me apologise again later.

(Melissa)

Melissa described her father sarcastically calling her 'such a princess' when she refused to do the babysitting, implying selfishness and self-importance, and went on to say how she was later forced to apologise for her behaviour. She described many incidents like this, seeing them as having resulted in her apologising and feeling guilty all the time: 'now I say [sorry] all the time, I have put out other people, or I'm an inconvenience to people. Or I'm in the way, or I'm wasting other people's time'. Other women also mentioned accusations of 'selfishness', for example, Louise said that her father often called her 'a selfish bitch'. Thus, the idea that the women are selfish for not taking on traditional female roles was a not uncommon aspect of the emotional abuse described by the women. In a different permutation of being forced into caring for others, Catherine talked about having to care for her mentally ill mother who was also named as her abuser:

I always felt like I had to look after Mum. And she had so many issues; it wasn't just mental, it was – this is disgusting, but she had a lot of incontinence issues and that sort of thing and she just didn't look after herself. And just, I honestly had to wash my mum's sheets and that sort of stuff because I was so embarrassed if people would come over.... And she wasn't old, she wasn't an invalid, she was just lazy. It was disgusting and I – this sounds horrible, I hated my mum for the longest of times. It was only in the year before she passed away that I – I wasn't even in contact with her much before she passed away which obviously is awful still, but I slowly started to build that, not even build up love but reduce the hate that I felt.

(Catherine)

Catherine identified feelings of disgust, shame and hate towards her mother, but she also alluded to guilt about these feelings when she said that hating her mother 'sounds horrible' and that it was 'obviously awful' to not have been in contact before her death. Catherine went on to say in an apologetic way that she had started to 'reduce the hate' by the time her mother died. Framing Catherine's confession is the discourse of the dutiful daughter, which promotes the gendered social ideal that women will selflessly love and care for their relatives, especially parents, in spite of how they themselves have been treated. Carole also described being left to care for her abusive, mentally ill mother as the only daughter in the family, and both she and Catherine expressed a level of resentment at what they saw as an extraordinary imposition in the context of emotional abuse.

Damned if you do, damned if you don't: mixed messages and 'no win' femininities

A particularly distinctive aspect of many women's narratives of childhood emotional abuse involved mixed messages about themselves, their identities and what they were expected to achieve in life. Rebecca grew up in 1970s Australia, and her narrative captures aspects of that social milieu for young women and the mixed messages she received as part of what she sees as parental emotional abuse:

When my brothers and I became teenagers we became these rebellious, opinionated young people who had very, very different ideas from my Mum and Dad, who were very middle-class, conservative, conventional, right? And they just looked at us and went, 'Oh my God'. And with me, in particular, they went, 'You can't be like this. We have to mould you into who we want you to be because you've come from us'. I wasn't allowed to have a voice and I just got told by my father, who was very dominating and very controlling, 'Shut up and go to your bedroom', if [my opinion] differed from his.... They were both emotionally abusive, very undermining, very invalidating.

(Rebecca)

Rebecca described being especially denied a voice and controlled through her parents' view that, as a girl, 'we have to mould you into who we want you to be because you've come from us'. This situates her as the property of her parents rather than as an autonomous person in her own right, with her behaviour understood to reflect on the family in a way that a son's does not. Moreover, while Rebecca described engaging with the counter-culture of her generation and its values of sexual freedom, independence and choice, she talked about the anxiety caused by receiving completely different messages from her parents that were often delivered in a dismissive or critical way: 'Because I was the only girl, I got the messages of, "Oh don't worry about an education. You need to find a man to take care of you".' As such, she described significant confusion about her capacities and direction in life. Rose grew up in the much later period of the 2000s, but she too talked about being given mixed messages in an emotionally abusive way about the social expectations on her as a girl:

> So do they [my parents] want me to get married and have kids or do they want me to go study? I can't have both at the same time.... I think they think I can do both but in my head I can't go and do masters and have a kid you know be pregnant and do masters ... they want it right now so I had two jobs and uni so I was working 35 hours a week and doing uni and it wasn't good enough.
>
> (Rose)

Rose presented herself as simply not knowing what her parents want from her because she believes they want her to 'have a kid ... right now' but also to complete her studies. However, for Rose, marriage and studies cannot take place at the same time and, as a consequence, she experiences her efforts at university and in her job as 'not good enough'. She therefore cannot win: whatever she does, she will be failing to fulfil inherently contradictory social expectations. Unlike Rebecca, Rose described mixed messages within the family itself while Rebecca received one set of messages in the family and another from outside it, reflecting the different historical contexts of their narratives. However, like Rebecca, Rose also depicted emotional abuse as causing high levels of stress and frustration for her, as well as anxiety and a range of psychosomatic complaints such as breathing difficulties and headaches. Emotional abuse therefore plays out in both Rebecca and Rose's narratives around wider contradictory discourses about femininity and women's place in the world. For Melissa, tensions about social expectations revolved more around the highly traditional Christian discourses subscribed to by her father as against her own desires as a contemporary young woman to complete school, get a higher education and have a career:

> My brother basically got his girlfriend knocked up at 17 and they had their first kid then and then they had to move out of home – my Dad saw him as becoming a man – he had to step up to a mark, whereas I moved out of home because I wanted to finish high school and go to university and that's disobedient to God's law apparently because I was meant to get married and have lots of children and that's just not my desire at all. So we've moved further apart.
>
> (Melissa)

The conflict between Melissa's goals for herself and those of her father have resulted in a level of estrangement from her family. April, who struggles with anorexia, also described receiving mixed messages about dependence versus independence. She talked about how she started to develop 'my own personality' during adolescence, and how her mentally ill mother 'just wanted me to be like a little girl forever because she could control me':

> I started to sort of develop my own personality, like differentiate. So I started to like my music and wanted to choose my own clothes. And I think for my Mum that was really hard because I think she just wanted me to be like a little girl forever because she could control me. So, yeah, that was sort of the beginning of abuse.
>
> (April)

April therefore described physical and emotional abuse as triggered by her efforts to become independent. In each of these cases, then, mixed messages revolved around gender discourses about independence versus dependence, or autonomy versus caring for others, sometimes more explicitly framed around marriage and children versus career. Louise's description of her experiences of receiving mixed messages was highly complex and distinctive from the others because it took place in the context of severe physical, sexual and emotional abuse from her father. She described her father buying gifts for her, on the one hand, and then accusing her of selfishness on the other. Much of Louise's father's behaviour is portrayed as manipulative, bribing her with gifts as part of grooming her for sexual abuse at the hands of himself and his friends. This grooming also involved significant levels of gas-lighting,[1] maternal alienation[2] and silencing, which resulted in years of denial of the sexual abuse by the rest of her family. However, in addition to silencing and denial of sexual abuse, Louise placed a heavy emphasis on the pernicious impact of her father's emotional abuse in and of itself because it resulted in 'not knowing whether I was good or bad or [if] what I was doing was OK'. As she said, it was 'that constant tension of "I don't know what's OK and I don't know what I can be, who I can be, what I can tell you, what I can't tell you"'. Louise described the uncertainty these experiences wrought, where she asks herself 'is this me? Is that me? No, hang on, no!' Louise then went on to explain how the emotional, physical and sexual abuse manifested in dissociative identity disorder (DID). DID can involve the emergence of multiple personalities (Briere and Runtz, 1993), and this is what Louise experiences:

> I don't know where I stand and one minute I can be really confident and the next minute I'm really shy because I think that I'm a piece of shit, kind of that sort of moving between the two quite....
>
> Q: Contradictory?
> A: Yeah, messages that I was getting.... I think in one sense, the DID's almost like a magnification of that sense. I've got some alters who are

highly confident, have no memories of abuse, have only good memories of my childhood, have – and all that kind of stuff, super confident, super able to get on stage, able to do whatever.

(Louise)

Thus, for Louise, DID rests on contradiction – on 'not knowing where I stand'. She told me that some of her alter personalities are highly confident and unaware of the abuse, and others are aware of the abuse and very emotionally distressed and self-harming. Louise understands the DID, and her anorexia and other self-harming behaviours, as having saved her rather than as symptomatic of psychopathology, describing a process of getting to know her alters and slowly coming to terms with the reality of sexual, physical and emotional abuse that has been denied in her family. One of the other women, Vanessa, also talked about being cowed into silence by her parents' denial of her and her sister's sexual abuse at the hands of their maternal grandfather, and she sees this as a significant aspect of her emotional abuse and as core to the severe and sudden panic disorder she later developed in young adulthood. For Louise, Vanessa and Aisha, then, emotional abuse was very much tied up with the gendered 'head fuck' of sexual abuse and sexual assault for girls (Warner, 2009).

A final feature of the emotional abuse described by the women was that it was often talked about as never ending, with many experiencing ongoing abuse from their families well into adulthood. Doyle (2001) also found that emotional abuse often persists beyond childhood and adolescence, unlike most physical and sexual abuse. For example, Melissa talked about how her father continues to criticise her and ignore her achievements at university, while Louise continues to experience manipulation and gas-lighting from her father, who has not faced up to his abuse. Rebecca continued to experience emotional abuse into her forties, at which time she issued her parents with an ultimatum about treating her with respect or 'I'm out of here and you will never see me again'. Some women, such as Catherine, Melissa, Louise, Aisha and Carole, talked about largely ceasing contact with their families because of continuing abuse. Where there was sexual abuse as well, there has usually been no proper recognition from abusers nor acknowledgement of silencing, denial and blame by non-offending parents. Some of the women whose abusers were their fathers, brothers, grandfathers or, later, their partners, described having developed a distrust and dislike of men. For example, Melissa said 'I hated all men.... I really, really hated them'. On the other hand, some women also described finding loving, intimate relationships with women or men who have been central to their recoveries, as well as other supportive friendships. Others placed an enormous emphasis on the importance of their children and the positive, non-abusive relationships they have been able to forge with them. For many of the women, then, developing positive, non-abusive relationships was central to overcoming the effects of abuse and this is explored further in Chapter 8.

In summary, the gendered dimensions of emotional abuse described by the women traversed three main spheres: the surveillance and control of the female body and sexuality; the enforcement of domestic and caring duties; and contradictory messages about self, identity and achievement. Gendered discourses that were part of this included those about female sexuality as dangerous, evil and the cause of rape; the positioning of women as sexualised body-objects; and the positioning of women as servicers of others' needs, including discourses about dutiful versus selfish daughters. These discourses, in turn, were linked in the women's accounts to intrusive and controlling practices of surveillance, confinement, emotional manipulation and verbal denigration. For some women, emotional abuse was specifically tied up with the manipulation, silencing, denial and victim-blaming that is so often part and parcel of sexual abuse and sexual assault for girls and women. Emotional abuse was also framed by more contemporary gender contradictions where women are expected to be independent, educated, responsible and self-determining persons but also responsible for the care of others (Turner, 1992). I now turn to the men's narratives of childhood emotional abuse in order to explore the different ways that gender discourses framed their understandings and experiences.

Men and childhood emotional abuse: 'becoming a man' in contexts of abuse

The men's narratives included a number of themes that revolved around a discourse about how to 'become a man' in the context of emotional abuse. Two of the men identified their fathers as their main abusers, describing abuse focused on stereotypically masculine areas of endeavour such as sports, work, studies and 'mates', meaning popularity with other men. For these two men, emotional abuse also involved stories of 'vanquishing the father', characterised by tales of eventually prevailing over and even defeating abusive fathers. As part of this, the men talked about becoming a 'better man' than their fathers. While the other two men were not particularly abused by their fathers, their narratives included not dissimilar themes of prevailing over abuse and of developing special talents and abilities because of their experiences, including emotional control and detachment from others. I will therefore show that while the childhood emotional abuse described by men involves highly gendered dimensions, as it does for women, the men drew on hegemonic masculinities to manage and prevail over its effects. Thus, I will show how these gendered discourses and practices enabled the men to frame emotional abuse and its consequences in quite distinctive ways from the women within narratives that were relatively free of the contradictions about gender and selfhood that so dogged the women's accounts. This is in part because, in Western cultures, there are fewer questions around what is valued in a man, and the men's narratives therefore reflected more hegemonic, less contradictory ideas about manhood and its unproblematic relationship to personhood. In contrast, the women's narratives were often founded on contradiction and on fundamentally problematic relationships between femininity and personhood.

Before teasing out the above themes, I want to first draw attention to two other important ways that the men's narratives differed from the women's. First, most of the men talked about themselves as *men* rather than as persons, that is, they named themselves as men, talked about growing into men, talked about how to be 'good' or 'better' men. In the men's narratives, then, a person *is* a man and a man *is* a person. Thus, personhood is *male*, so contemporaneous with each other as to require no explanation. The women never named themselves as women nor talked about growing into 'good' or 'better' women: they talked about themselves only in the more gender neutral terms of 'persons'. This is interesting, because it has been argued within feminist theory that women can never appear as non-gendered subjects (Weedon, 1987). Yet in participants' own talk about themselves, it is the men who present themselves in heavily gendered terms, not the women, and as the analysis progresses, the discourses driving this and the related gender practices will become evident. Second, the men tended to portray themselves as realising from a relatively early age that they were not to blame for the abuse they endured and that, instead, the problem lay entirely with their abusers. Thus, the men tended to place responsibility wholly with their abusers, not with themselves and, as a result, there was no talk of guilt or self-blame. Along these lines, Lachlan described coming to realise by adolescence that his father was 'actually a fairly angry guy, but I still could never really challenge the notion that it was his own doings that led him there'. He also talked about establishing what he calls a 'manly bond' with his younger brother, who was not abused, and how together they supported each other in the view that their father was fully to blame:

> [It is] very important to the healing to know that your sibling, who's actually seen you go through that can say, 'bro I know how much you went through and you didn't do anything wrong, you know, he's got massive issues and he could never be the father that we've longed for, but that's okay because we can be better men than that'.
>
> (Lachlan)

This begins to hint at this idea of striving to be 'a better man' than the abusive father, which I will come to later. Paul described trying to please his emotionally abusive, alcoholic father by working hard at school. When he brought home a positive school report, his father failed to acknowledge it. He said:

> And then something just clicked inside my head. It was just 'you're wasting your time'. It doesn't matter what you do he's never ever going to see he's proud of you – whether he is or not is irrelevant – he will never ever see he's proud of you of what you've done. It doesn't matter if you get dux [top pupil] of the school it will make no difference. He will not say that he is proud of you. So then I felt fine at school.... Because I had no reason to try any more.
>
> (Paul)

Thus, Paul described realising that his father would never be proud of him, and he simply gave up trying at that point. Ben largely experienced race-based abuse from peers at school because of his Asian heritage, but he also talked about his white stepfather's lack of empathy and victim-blaming response to this:

> But he told me, he said 'What did you do? You must have done something wrong'. And I just looked at him like, what would you know, you're one of them anyway. [I] went to my room and I had this epiphany, sat in my room and I said 'Well, you come here alone and you leave alone and stuff just happens in the middle' you know? And I was 12.
>
> (Ben)

Ben described himself as realising at 12 years of age that he was completely alone in dealing with the abuse, dismissing and rejecting his stepfather as 'one of them anyway' as well as taking up the philosophical attitude of 'you come here alone and you leave alone'. Thus, for Ben, it was *contra mundum* – him against the world – in part reflecting his lonely experience of racial abuse in a predominantly white community but also masculinity discourses about separateness and detachment from others. I will now move on to explore how two of the men depicted emotional abuse as concerned with the stereotypically masculine endeavours of sport, work, studies and mates.

My dad's favourite sport

Lachlan described experiencing significant abuse from his father in relation to playing football, his father's 'favourite game'. Lachlan admitted that in spite of excelling at football, he did not very much enjoy it, particularly as he got older and developed other interests, but he did not feel he had much choice in the matter. However, the time came when he wanted to give it up:

> With any other parent I think that they'd say, do what you want to do, and this turned into a very, very big problem, which I think this is where the abuse actually really started big time.... I wanted to stop playing football. My father acted like an absolute animal for a couple of years and he actually didn't let me stop.... It was all about him.... I got tonsillitis, right?... [and he was] using profanities and things like that, he forced me to go ... the way that he treated me was like a dog, almost like, you know, he just wanted me to play, he didn't care that I was [sick] ... he was just really cold towards me, like a dog [that] we assume doesn't really have the emotions that a human being does that are really complex.... He wasn't being a father, basically.... No empathy whatsoever. And that is only one example. And I think that example pretty much illustrates that many other things that he did were along those lines. It was all about him because of his dissatisfaction with his life, led to out-lashing on other people, particularly me, being the eldest son it often just came out on me.
>
> (Lachlan)

Lachlan described being treated 'like a dog' that 'doesn't really have the emotions that a human being does'. There is a strong sense in this account of having been dehumanised through lack of empathy from his father and thereby treated like an animal. However, again, this is clearly understood to be his father's problem because of his 'dissatisfaction with his own life', leading him to live through his son and his successes. Lachlan therefore understands his father's abuse as a projection and 'reflection of his own worthlessness to himself' rather than any reflection on him. Most importantly, though, there is a sense that he has rights as a human being and that his father's abuse fundamentally transgressed those rights: in this sense, then, his father's abusive behaviour is understood as morally wrong.

Work, mates and being the man

Paul's narrative positioned much of the emotional and physical abuse he and his brothers experienced at the hands of their father as concerned with success and failure in the worlds of work, study and mates. Paul's family was working class, migrating from Britain to Australia in the 1960s when he was a child, and his narrative is powerfully framed by this historical class background. He first explains why he was particularly singled out for abuse by his father:

> I was the least powerful and the lowest peg in the household too and everyone made sure that I knew that – even my brothers made sure that I knew that I was the bottom of the rung and they were the strong ones and so I retreated basically within myself. I became much of a people pleaser … that was my defensive mechanism – I figured if people like me they won't hurt me, and it didn't work out.… But the thing of course I thought that would make people like me wasn't what fitted on my dad's thing because you had to be a tough guy to be a friend with my dad and I was not a tough guy – I was the baby of the family.
>
> (Paul)

Paul described the household in hierarchical terms, with himself on 'the lowest peg' and his mother entirely excluded, even though she was actually the bread-winner because of his father's alcoholism. It was therefore a quintessentially male hierarchy, with his father at the top. Paul believes he was abused by his father because 'I was not a tough guy' and, in order to cope, he described becoming a 'people pleaser', a lesser, feminised identity that he acknowledged was never going to placate his father. Paul went on to describe the nature of his father's attacks on his sons:

> The thing about my dad is – I won't say never but he wasn't physically violent on a lot of occasions but enough to keep you scared. And he would threaten it – like he used to say 'I don't smack my kids – I punch them with the fist' … he would give us lectures … he would berate you, he would call you – he would tell you that you are never ever going to amount to

nothing.... All you're going to be is a labourer – this was his way of encouraging you to study hard and get a job.... And his favourite phrase was 'You are nothing' and he would usually say it at the top of his voice two inches away from you – nose to nose.

(Paul)

Paul portrayed his father's abuse as focused on the idea that he and his brothers were going to be failures and would 'never ever amount to nothing – all you're going to be is a labourer', framed within discourses of masculinity that centre work and achievement, and working-class discourses of personal failure, inadequacy, lack of intelligence and limited aspirations. However, like Lachlan, Paul explained his father's accusations of impending failure as very much a function of projecting of his own sense of worthlessness and failure onto him rather than deficiencies in himself:

He had no self-esteem of his own because he had ruined his life and he knew it through the drinking.... And his way of getting any self-esteem because he couldn't build himself up – was ... [to] level the playing field because if I'm here and they're [the sons are] down here.... I'll pull them down ... but of course, typical of an alcoholic, his friends thought he was the best thing out under the sun. Oh he was fantastic.

(Paul)

Paul went on to explain how his father had to be 'the man':

He's got to be the man. And he used to boast about us kids in front of his mates. He had to sit there, because he used to take us down the pub but he had to babysit us because mum was working and he wasn't – he would take us to the pub and you had to sit there and listen to him brag on you to his friends and you're thinking 'But when I get home you're going to call me useless and an idiot and beat me up' and you think.... And that was so hard because you couldn't say anything to him.

(Paul)

Thus, Paul sees his father's behaviour as pathetic, 'bragging' to his friends about his sons and then calling Paul 'useless and an idiot' at home. He said: 'for him to encourage you, to say you can study ... would mean that he was saying that you were better than him and he couldn't do that'. Thus, the abuse is depicted as fundamentally competitive, where the father must prevail and be superior to, and better than, the sons. He added that his father could not acknowledge when Paul won an apprenticeship, the pinnacle of success in his father's eyes, saying how 'it was more like "I've told you that you're not going to get an achievement, now you've gone and got one ... you can't do that to me"'. Paul's father is now dead and he muses, 'I wonder how he would go now?' given that Paul has almost finished a university degree. He goes on to say that the abuse left him with feelings of fear that he was 'not going to be successful' and an enduring 'fear of authority'. More than this, though, Paul suffered a major psychological crisis after a series of workplace accidents when he was around 40 years old, triggering severe panic, depression and suicide attempts that he now believes emanated from his father's emotional abuse. Perhaps it is unsurprising, given the focus of the abuse on success at work, that this crisis was triggered in a workplace context.

Controlling emotion

Another way that discourses of masculinity were brought to bear in the abuse described by the men was through the idea of learning to control their emotions and their bodies. Ben said that he would 'shut down' in response to the abuse but, inside, it would be 'a big ball of fire' that he would 'condense' and that 'it would be red ... the red would be hot and then.... I'd just [go] like "grrrrr"'. Thus, Ben would be angry but he would push this feeling down until it later erupted. Henry was emotionally and sexually abused by his older sister and he explained how he taught himself to deal with his feelings towards her by plunging his hand into scalding hot water:

> I remember one thing I kept doing when I was younger was I would fill the bathroom sink up with like really hot water and stick my hand in it, and I found that the longer you could hold your hand in the water, the more control you had over yourself, and therefore the more control you could have over your emotions. So, I basically managed to shut off most of my emotions until I was about 22, 23, ish.
>
> (Henry)

Like Louise earlier, Henry called this self-harming practice 'dissociation from my feelings' but it is quite different to Louise's account of self-harm and dissociation. Louise presented herself as seeking to repress and communicate feelings of hurt and guilt through harming herself, whereas Henry depicted self-harm as way of gaining mastery over his emotions. Henry went on to describe himself as 'sociopathic' and as having developed violent sexual dreams because of the emotional and sexual abuse. He said 'the violent impulses sort of progressively got worse, and then.... I kept going, yeah no, I'm not going to turn around and belt that fuckwit [my sister], and eventually [it] just started ... my dreams instead'. Thus, the dreams are understood to have started because he repressed his urges to be physically violent towards his sister, although he did use violence against her to stop the abuse once he had grown bigger than her. Below, he explained how he began to use drugs to suppress the violent dreams:

> Well, one of the reasons I started smoking weed when I was near the end of high school is because of the dreams I kept having. I understood the theory behind, or the idea or whatever behind having sex dreams, like as a release and a cathartic thing. My dreams were like something out of Friday the 13th.

Q: OK, so quite violent?

A: Quite violent, very, very vivid and realistic. And I never woke up with like a hard-on or anything like that, but I did always feel calm, relaxed and happy the next morning.

Q: OK, so they didn't leave you with feelings of fear or, you know, discomfort?

A: No, I quite enjoyed them. I quite enjoyed them, which is why I started smoking weed because it stopped me dreaming.

Q: OK, so why did you want to stop them then, if they had a relaxing effect?

A: Because I kind of wanted to do it while I was awake.

Q: OK, so, how did that make you feel?

A: Like it was a really bad fucking idea.

Q: So did that frighten you or concern you?

A: Yeah, more concern than frightened because I didn't want to – well, it's not like I didn't want to kill people around me it's more that I didn't want to suffer the consequences thereof.

(Henry)

As can be seen above, I probed further into what it was that made Henry want to suppress the dreams, and he said that it was because he did not want to 'suffer the consequences' of killing rather than because he saw it as wrong or upsetting to hurt people. He expanded on this by adding that he would 'never feel a drop of guilt' if he had acted:

It's not something I'm going to go and do. I mean I know I could do it and never feel a drop of guilt about it, or anything like that.

Q: Really?

A: Yeah.

Q: Explain that.

A: I don't know.

Q: How do you know that you wouldn't feel a drop of guilt?

A: Because I've imagined doing it and just ... go cool, what would this feel like to do that – nope, wouldn't care ... so I'm pretty sure I could do it and not care, but it's not something I'm going to go and do.

(Henry)

This lack of empathy, guilt or remorse is in in part why Henry sees himself as sociopathic, and why his psychologist agrees with this diagnosis. Henry's dreams and impulses are now under control through treatment, as is the ongoing depression he experiences. Ben also talked about how he learned to 'shut out' things in his life as if 'switches go off and on'. Related to this, he also talked about learning how to get what he needed from people in a very instrumental way because of the abuse:

And this idea of positive attitude had started, you know, from quite young because I'd also [latched] onto people who would have said something which gave a [positive attitude] – because I didn't have a father. Well I did, my step father but he didn't really say much at all ... but what I used to do was I used to take what I needed, and what I wanted and I was very aware what I was doing, very aware.... Even if it's just one thing a day from one person. I see people as Lego and I would just take the piece that I need. You see and when I was ... and I would then build up my idea about what a man should be.

Q: You'd take the bits that were useful to you?
A: Yeah exactly.

(Ben)

Ben said that he 'sees people as Lego and I would just take the piece that I needed'. Thus, people are portrayed as objects that he uses to get his needs met, seeing himself as entitled to do this because 'I didn't have a father' and this allowed him to 'then build up my idea about what a man should be'. Thus, Ben depicted a calculated process of drawing on others in order to 'become a man' in the absence of a father figure, and positioned himself as entirely aware and in control of what he was doing. He went on to say, similarly to Henry, that he feels 'very emotionless within relationships' and that 'relationships don't need to be that high on the hierarchy' for him:

Well, what happened recently I had – and this is part of my makeup now, you know, whether it comes from this abuse earlier on or not feeling I had a father – all these sorts of things. But I feel very emotionless within my – in some areas for some reason, I don't know what it is. It's mainly relationships, I really don't feel anything.

(Ben)

Ben also called many of the women he had had relationships with 'just too much hard work'. Ben therefore presented himself as quite detached from others, including his female partners. While both Ben and Henry described their abuse-related lack of emotion as bringing certain advantages through detachment from others, their narratives also involved a level of concern that this was not 'normal', with Ben in particular hoping that he could have successful intimate relationships in the future.

Vanquishing the father and being a better man

As noted earlier, the narratives from the two men whose fathers were their abusers involved a more specific discourse of 'vanquishing the father' and 'being a better man' than him. Paul mused earlier about how his father might now see him if he were alive, given that he has almost completed a university degree. He also talked with some satisfaction about reaching a greater age than his father, and having earned much more money and being much more successful in his work than his father:

> They weren't turning points but they were the best moments in my life in regards to my father – one was when I turned 50 because he didn't make it that far and when I – and I realised this – and I didn't do the maths until later when I was at university but I realised when I left work I was earning in excess of five times what he would have ever earned in the best years of his life. There was a time difference there – not that much. And I was over $120,000 running my own business profit – didn't pay tax on it all but that's what we worked out – that's what our income was equal to – it was about $120,000 that my wife and I were earning in our business when I got sick, so that was 10–15 years ago so that was a decent amount of money … not so much now but in those days it was big money…. But I worked out my dad probably never got over $20,000 in his entire life…. It still would be three or four times of what he got … and now…. Well this [time at university] is my second time to succeed.
>
> (Paul)

Thus, for Paul, surpassing his father 'were the best moments in my life'. Paul also talked about his Christianity and the leadership role he has taken at his church in helping others to manage their lives as part of his success in life. Lachlan's narrative similarly drew on this discourse of vanquishing his father. He went on to describe how once he had grown in size, 'it got to a point where he knew, like almost like a coward, he would intimidate me physically and would hit me when I was younger, but as I got older it was like, "Do you want to go?" you know? I don't think so, not any more', until matters eventually came to a head:

> As I was finishing year 12 things got really bad between myself and my father, simply because as I was getting more intelligent and becoming more open to how the world actually is and how adults should behave, I realised that what he's doing is just not on … because of [my studies] my eyes were being opened to the world and I realised that my father's got big, big problems. And it was at that stage where I was almost – it was a desperate attempt on my behalf to try to challenge him to make him see his wrongs, but he would always battle me and defend his position.
>
> Q: So you were starting to buck up against each other?
> A: Oh, locking horns all the time … [he would say things] to me and I'm absolutely, completely innocent and I haven't done anything. I think, [I] just snapped…. So we got into a bit of a fight, and then the day after, I think it continued on and locking horns over something, and then he threatened me and he said, 'oh' you know, 'I'll put your head through the wall', or whatever and I'm like, 'Yeah, well fucking bring it on', you know, 'do you want to go?' … I was, I'm 18 at that time.

Q: So you're fully grown?

A: Oh yeah, bigger than I am now, because of sport and things like that, and that's not right behaviour. That's not, you should never, ever resort to physical violence to solve your problems, but it's like the father against son, things just blow out of proportion sometimes and, ultimately it's the father's responsibility, but he doesn't, he's incapable of dealing with things on a proper level.

(Lachlan)

Lachlan talked about 'locking horns' with his father, drawing on the analogy of stags in the wild fighting for supremacy, and how it was 'the father against the son' because his father was 'incapable of dealing with things'. Lachlan again positioned himself as 'completely innocent' and undeserving of his father's verbal abuse, presenting himself as effectively stepping into the corrective, parental role, judging his father's behaviour and striving 'to make him see his wrongs'. However, he also retaliated physically because he had grown taller and stronger than his father. He went on to say that his father later apologised to him, but that:

His apologies were never really the apologies that I wanted. I wanted him to be proactive and be a man and be a father and come before me and confess that he made mistakes and he's not proud of them but he's going to work towards being a better man, and I never got that. It was almost like a submissive defeated apology.

(Lachlan)

Lachlan said that he wanted his father to take responsibility for himself but, instead, his apologies were 'like a submissive, defeated apology'. Thus, Lachlan wanted his father to 'be proactive and be a man and be a father' but instead Lachlan found himself positioned as the victor, which was not what he wanted. He went on to say that he has become a Christian and has forgiven his father: 'I'm working towards slowly just forgiving him and trying to maintain some kind of contact with him, even though our relationship can't be what I would hope for, as a son to a father.' Further to the idea of vanquishing the father, Lachlan also talked about 'being a better man' than his father has been. A little similarly to Ben earlier, Lachlan asked himself in the absence of a positive father figure, 'what is it to be a man?', constructing his father as 'the appearance of a man' rather than a 'real man'. He goes on to say that:

I do consider myself, actually, overall, fortunate to not only come out from my situation of abuse as a child but to actually.... I don't think I would have been the man that I am today if it were not for all the lessons that I've chosen to learn and gain from that abuse.

He went on to clarify that being a man means 'to be the leader, to be a teacher and to be strong' and 'to see things for what they are, to have the courage to admit your failures'. Lachlan also clarified that there are 'the soft skills of being a man', too, such as needing to be 'intimate, there are times that you have to put your pride away, listen to people, take what they have to say seriously, be empathetic to their emotions'. Thus, being a proper, 'real' man is constructed as being a well-rounded individual who is both strong and empathic to others, this emphasis on empathy perhaps reflecting the lack of this quality in Lachlan's experiences with his father. In answer to my question about whether women can also have these qualities, he said that they 'can be just as strong as men are' but that:

> It is important that a woman knows that she can actually fall back onto her man if she needs to. That he can be, you know, like the rock that if she's having difficulties in her life, she's got a soft place to fall.
>
> Q: And so, do you see that as more ... of the man's responsibility, perhaps than hers?
> A: I do think so.
>
> (Lachlan)

He said that his views come at least in part from seeing 'all the women in my family having to be the leaders and being stressed and having to deal with incompetent men',[3] but he also described his realisation that his girlfriend is more emotionally vulnerable than him. He went on to say that 'men are given certain qualities that help them be there ... they stem from the primal qualities of like being able to shut certain parts of your mind off when you need to deal with problems'. Thus, Lachlan drew on a discourse of natural gender difference that positions men as more rational and as better able to control their bodies and emotions than women (Connell, 2005). Moreover, like Henry and Ben earlier, Lachlan understands himself as having gained an additional advantage in this regard through his experiences of abuse. Ben went further than this, saying, 'I think I've nearly walked the path of destiny and I think that [it] was one of these instances that if I couldn't handle it, it might not have come'. Thus, he believes that he was abused because he is especially strong and he went on to say how he has gone on to 'champion the underdog' and has adopted aspects of Buddhism to 'teach people how to be positive'. Further to this, Ben described how he now interacts with others as a result of this learning:

> If there was my child there and someone decided to give her a smack on the hand about grabbing something and it's not their child, you know, I'm not going to throw the table but I will stand up there and I will tell you in no uncertain terms, using my eyes and using my tone of voice, because it's a practiced technique, and tell you that you're just not to do that ever again and that will be it because you know I've always been [through my work], the three Cs, clear, concise and correct. When I speak to you, this is how I'm going to speak to you and because I need it done like this, like that – OK?
>
> (Ben)

Thus, Ben sees the abuse he experienced as enabling him to learn particularly well how to command authority, using his body through the tone of his voice and eye contact in his interactions with others. In summary, then, the men's narratives of emotional abuse involved significantly gendered dimensions that included locating blame entirely with their abusers and not themselves; abuse focused on stereotypically masculine areas of endeavour such as sporting achievement, work, studies and mates; learning to master their emotions through self-control; vanquishing abusive fathers and other abusers, including the use of physical violence when they had grown; and becoming 'better men', which included becoming leaders and teachers in order to guide others, taking responsibility for themselves, exercising empathic skills, and being authoritative and in control. These gendered dimensions of emotional abuse draw on hegemonic masculinity discourses that construct idealised manhood in particular ways, with abuse constructed as providing a special, alternative pathway for learning how to become a man, usually in the absence of a positive father figure. However, while Henry's narrative included the masculinity practices of controlling emotion and using physical force, it also differed from the others because he lives with what he calls sociopathy. There is not space here to elaborate this further, but because Henry experiences a quite extreme level of emotional detachment, as well as sexually violent fantasies, his narrative involved less celebration of masculinity than the others and a more obvious struggle with identity and depression. I now turn to examine the differences between the women's and men's narratives in more detail, showing how childhood emotional abuse can be understood as a powerful tool of engendering in everyday life.

Entrenching gender binaries through childhood emotional abuse

I want to reiterate here that in addition to highly gendered descriptions of childhood emotional abuse, participants also talked about emotional abuse in the non-gendered terms outlined earlier: I have purposively and selectively focused on the gendered aspects of their experiences because no other research into childhood emotional abuse to date has explicitly done so, in spite of the fact that findings from other studies point to its importance (Downs and Miller, 1998; Harper and Arias, 2004). The above analysis has therefore demonstrated that women's and men's narratives of childhood emotional abuse include gendered dimensions that have a number of implications, including for how individuals might manage the impact of abuse in their lives. First, the men's narratives revolved around a discourse about how to be 'a better man' in spite of abuse, and this included the development of self-control – especially control of emotion, emotional detachment, rationality and the use of power and authority. What emerged as so distinctive in the men's narratives was how manhood, constructed through a hegemonic discourse of masculinity, was usually conceived of as a unitary and fundamentally good thing, so commensurate with being a 'good person' that this underlying assumption need not be stated. Thus, to be 'a good man' was something worth striving for, bringing positive self-identity for most of the men and advantages in managing other people. Male bodies were also in this picture through the use of physical force to vanquish abusers and in gaining mastery over emotion. Moreover, conceptualisations of being a good man sometimes rested on assumptions about women as naturally more emotional and vulnerable than men, and as therefore requiring leadership, protection or, in one case, avoidance. Thus, hegemonic masculinities in the men's narratives at times relied on a particular understanding of femininity as different from and lesser than masculinity: contemporary gender theorists point out that hegemonic masculinities often rely on devaluation of, and distancing from, the feminine (Connell, 2005). While hegemonic masculinities were quite central in the men's narratives, it is important to be aware, though, that this is unlikely to reflect the real complexities or changing nature of masculinities in these men's lives more generally. Moreover, in men accounting for childhood emotional abuse, it is quite likely that questions of masculinity might become particularly important because they have been disempowered through their positioning as victims: it is women who are more commonly thought of as 'natural victims', not men.

There was simply no counterpart to the 'better man' discourse for the women, who talked about themselves in non-gendered terms while often depicting highly gendered practices of shaming, guilt, manipulation and control based on contradictory femininities that undermined personhood. More specifically, the discourses framing these practices not uncommonly constructed two conflicting femininities, one idealised and one not. For example, the women were positioned as sexual, disgusting and culpable against non-sexual and blameless; as fat instead of thin; as slovenly as against clean and tidy; and as selfish rather than selfless. Thus, there was usually more than one version of femininity in play in the narratives at any one time, one 'good' and the other 'bad' (and often sexualised), with these binaries embedded in long-standing historical discourses about women and the feminine (MacSween, 1993). Further to this, some of the emotional abuse was also framed by other more contemporary contradictions about women as either 'for others' or 'for themselves', that is, as dependent carers of others or independent, autonomous women. This is a well-recognised tension in contemporary femininities that positions women simultaneously as persons, with all the rights and entitlements that go with Western conceptions of individuality, and as non-persons in the service of others (see Turner, 1992). These tensions and contradictions are experienced to some extent by all women, but the above analysis shows how they can be dramatically brought to life in childhood emotional abuse to produce powerful feelings of worthlessness, anxiety, guilt, confusion, shame, and a sense of not being able to win either way. Indeed, shame in particular has been shown to be an especially gendered emotion (Probyn, 2005) and this is explored further in terms of the relationship between abuse, shame and eating disorders in the next chapter. Thus, childhood emotional abuse in a number of women's narratives captured a host of gender contradictions about self and selfhood undercut by long-standing negative discourses about the feminine and the female body as something to be controlled and repressed.

In terms of the women's narratives, then, there was no discourse about being a 'good or better woman' because 'femininity' and 'womanhood' often carry with them a host of potentially negative meanings and practices that undermine personhood and socially valued identities.[4] And while the women also had access to other seemingly gender-neutral discourses about themselves as auto-nomous persons, these are based on masculinist assumptions about personhood and autonomy that sit in some tension with femininity discourses (Burman, 1996), contributing to a theme in the narratives of being to some extent 'damned if you do and damned if you don't'. Perhaps somewhat obviously, then, there is no 'better woman' discourse in the narratives because there is no 'hegemonic femininity', reflecting not only the fact that contemporary femininities are highly contradictory but also that women continue to be subjugated in gender power relations. As such, then, contradictory and subjugated femininities often left the women with the impression that there was something fundamentally wrong with *them*, and many talked of struggling to find a positive sense of themselves for many years after abuse. In contrast, while childhood emotional abuse was also distressing for the men, their access to hegemonic masculinities enabled them to construct abuse as unwarranted and as an assault on their human rights that was largely reflective of the weakness and wrongness of their abusers, in some cases juxtaposing their abusers against idealised, hegemonic versions of masculinity and finding them wanting.

Because this research is qualitative and the sample is small, it cannot make claims about the prevalence of mental health problems between the women and the men as a result of these gender discourses and practices. However, it was certainly the case that in line with aspects of Harper and Arias' (2004) findings, many more of the women described struggling with so-called internalising prob-lems of anxiety, depression, eating disorders, self-harm, dissociation and feel-ings of shame, guilt and self-blame, and while these were less of a feature in the men's narratives, so-called externalising practices of emotional detachment and anger towards abusers were common. There is evidence that individuals who attribute maltreatment to factors external to themselves do better than those who attribute it to internal factors, such as rejection of themselves as 'bad' people (Doyle, 2001). What this analysis shows is how processes of attribution are framed by gendered social discourses and related practices and that these risk entrenching binaries of gender along relatively traditional lines.

These findings have implications for how we as practitioners approach helping and supporting women and men who are struggling with mental health problems as a result of childhood emotional abuse. Most importantly, they draw attention to the need to consider gender, as well as race and class, when working with individuals. I explore in some detail in Chapter 8 how practitioners might bring a socially informed perspective to their work that engages with gender. I want to re-emphasise here, though, that the gender binaries apparent from this analysis of childhood emotional abuse narratives do not necessarily reflect the wider complexities of these women's and men's lives in relation to gender. In contemporary societies, gender and gender relations are shifting and highly complex (Connell, 2005), framed by unstable and contradictory discourses. However, it is important to be aware that gender can be quite central to childhood emotional abuse, and that how it plays out will also ebb and flow over time as what it means to be a girl or boy, woman or man, shifts along with other social positionings in relation to class and race. I have touched a little here on how gender frames aspects of childhood emotional abuse for some women and men at this particular historical juncture. In the next chapter, I tease out in some detail how emotional, sexual and physical abuse can play out in the specific symptoms of eating disorders, conditions which are disproportionately diagnosed in women and girls who have been abused but for which explanatory frameworks remain highly contested and, outside of feminist research, persistently gender blind.

Notes

1 Gas-lighting is a type of psychological abuse that aims to make the victim doubt their own perceptions, memories and sanity. It is common in abuse, and involves selective omission of information, the twisting around of information and the presentation of false information (Domestic Violence Resource Centre Victoria, www.dvrcv.org.au/knowledge-centre/our-blog/gaslighting-stalking-and-intimate-partner-violence, accessed 29 April 2015).
2 Maternal alienation involves dividing the mother and child from each other in gendered violence and abuse (Laing, 1999; Morris, 1999).
3 Lachlan described how his mother was the primary breadwinner because of his father's problems, and how his father also created significant maternal alienation between him and his mother when they divorced. He now has a close relationship with his mother based on his growing insight into his father's behaviour.
4 One exception to this was the feminine identity of motherhood, and many women talked about the pleasure and satisfaction they had had gained from loving and caring for their children, and not reproducing abuse. The two men who had children also emphasised the importance of loving, non-abusive relationships with their children. These participants therefore challenged the assumption of childhood abuse as necessarily re-enacted in subsequent generations.

References

Bell, S. (2011) Through a Foucauldian lens: a geneology of child abuse, *Journal of Family Violence*, 26, pp. 101–108.

Bernstein, D.P. and Fink, L. (1998) *Childhood Trauma Questionnaire: A Retrospective Self-Report*. San Antonio: The Psychological Corporation.

Boulton, S. and Hindle, D. (2000) Emotional abuse: the work of a multidisciplinary consultation group in a child psychiatric service. *Clinical Child Psychology and Psychiatry*, 5(3), pp. 439–452.

Bowlby, J. (1988) *A Secure Base: Clinical Applications of Attachment Theory*. London: Routledge.

Briere, J. and Runtz, M. (1993) Child sexual abuse, *Journal of Interpersonal Violence*, 8(3), pp. 312–330.

Burman, E. (1996) The spec(tac)ular economy of difference. In S. Wilkinson and C. Kitzinger (eds), *Representing the Other*. London: Sage Publications, pp. 138–140.

Coates, D. (2010) Impact of childhood abuse: biopsychosocial pathways through which adult mental health is compromised, *Australian Social Work*, 63(4), pp. 391–403.

Connell, R.W. (2005) *Masculinities*, second edition. Crows Nest: Allen & Unwin.

Downs, W.R. and Miller, B.A. (1998) Relationships between experiences of parental violence during childhood and women's psychiatric symptomatology, *Journal of Interpersonal Violence*, 13, pp. 438–457.

Downs, W.M. and Rindels, B. (2004) Adulthood depression, anxiety, and trauma symptoms: a comparison of women with nonabusive, abusive, and absent father figures in childhood, *Violence and Victims*, 19(6), pp. 659–671.

Doyle, C. (2001) Surviving and coping with emotional abuse in childhood, *Clinical Child Psychology and Psychiatry*, 6(3), pp. 387–402.

Gavey, N. (2005) *Just Sex? The Cultural Scaffolding of Rape*. Hove: Routledge.

Gavey, N. and Schmidt, J. (2011) 'Trauma of rape' discourse: a double-edged template for everyday understandings of the impact of rape? *Violence Against Women*, 17, pp. 433–456.

Glaser, D. (2002) Emotional abuse and neglect (psychological maltreatment): a conceptual framework. *Child Abuse & Neglect*, 26, pp. 697–714.

Harper, F.W.K. and Arias, I. (2004) The role of shame in predicting adult anger and depressive symptoms among victims of child psychological maltreatment, *Journal of Family Violence*, 19(6), pp. 367–375.

Hart, S.N., Germain, R.B. and Brassard, M.R. (eds) (1983) *Proceedings Summary of the International Conference on Psychological Abuse of Children and Youth*. Indiana University: Office for the Study of the Psychological Rights of the Child.

Kennedy, M.A., Ip, K., Samra, J. and Gorzalka, B.B. (2007) The role of childhood emotional abuse in disordered eating, *Journal of Emotional Abuse*, 7(1), pp. 17–36.

Krause, E.D., Mendelson, T. and Lynch, T.R. (2003) Childhood emotional invalidation and adult psychological distress: the mediating role of emotional inhibition, *Child Abuse and Neglect*, 27(2), pp. 199–213.

Laing, L. (1999) A different balance altogether? Incest offenders in treatment. In J. Breckenridge and L. Laing (eds), *Challenging Silence: Innovative Responses to Sexual and Domestic Violence*. Sydney: Allen & Unwin, pp. 137–152.

Maciejewski, P.K. and Mazure, C.M. (2006) Fear of critisicm and rejection mediates an association between childhood emotional abuse and adult onset of major depression, *Cognitive Therapy and Research*, 30(1), pp. 105–122.

McNay, L. (2004) Situated intersubjectivity. In B. Marshall and A. Witz (eds), *Engendering the Social: Feminist Encounters with Sociological Theory*. Maidenhead: Open University Press, pp. 171–186.

MacSween, M. (1993) *Anorexic Bodies*. London: Routledge.

May-Chahal, C. (2006) Gender and child maltreatment: the evidence base, *Social Work and Society*, 4(1), pp. 53–68.

Messman-Moore, T.L. and Garrigus, A.S. (2007) The association of child abuse and eating disorder symptomatology: the importance of multiple forms of abuse and revictimization, *Journal of Aggression, Maltreatment & Trauma*, 14(3), pp. 51–72.

Morris, A. (1999) Adding insult to injury, *Trouble & Strife*, 40, pp. 30–35.

Mullen, P.E., Martin, J.L., Anderson, J.C., Romans, S.E. and Herbison, G.C. (1996) The long-term impact of the physical, emotional and sexual abuse of children: a community study, *Child Abuse and Neglect*, 20(1), pp. 7–21.

O'Dougherty Wright, M., Crawford, E. and Del Castillo, D. (2009) Childhood emotional maltreatment and later psychological distress among college students: the mediating role of maladaptive schemas, *Child Abuse and Neglect*, 33, pp. 59–68.

Pelcovitz, D., Kaplan, S., Goldenberg, B., Mandel, F., Lehane, J. and Guarrera, J. (1994) Post-traumatic stress disorder in physically abused adolescents, *Journal of the American Academy of Child and Adolescent Psychiatry*, 33(3), pp. 305–312.

Probyn, E. (2005) *Blush: Faces of Shame*. Minneapolis: University of Minnesota Press.

Rorty, M. and Yager, J. (1996) Speculations on the role of childhood abuse in the development of eating disorders among women. In M.F. Schwartz and L. Cohn (eds), *Sexual Abuse and Eating Disorders*. New York: Brunner-Routledge, pp. 23–35.

Sachs-Ericsson, N., Gayman, M.D., Kendall-Tackett, K., Lloyd, D.A., Medley, A., Collins, N., Corsentino, E. and Sawyer, K. (2010) The long-term impact of childhood abuse on internalizing disorders among older adults: the moderating role of self-esteem, *Aging and Mental Health*, 14(4), pp. 489–501.

Thomas, S.P. and Hall, J.M. (2008) Life trajectories of female child abuse survivors thriving in adulthood, *Qualitative Health Research*, 18, pp. 149–166.

Turner, B. (1992) *Regulating Bodies: Essays in Medical Sociology*. London: Routledge.

Warner, S. (2009) *Understanding the Effects of Child Sexual Abuse: Feminist Revolutions in Theory, Research and Practice*. London: Routledge.

Weedon, C. (1987) *Feminist Practice and Poststructuralist Theory*. Oxford: Basil Blackwell.

5 Pleasure and pain

The management of abuse-related emotion in eating disorders

There has been growing attention over the past three decades to the presence of childhood abuse in the backgrounds of many women with eating disorders. As was pointed out in Chapter 2, there is evidence that sexual abuse and emotional abuse are common among women who experience eating disorders. In spite of this, there has been little systematic attention to how women themselves experience an eating disorder in contexts of abuse. This is in part because of historical resistance to acknowledging sexual abuse among women diagnosed with eating disorders on the part of powerful male psychiatrists (Wooley, 1994), and women's understandable reticence to disclose in this context. However, there is also a long history of pathologising the families of eating disordered women in ways that may well play down and obscure non-sexual forms of abuse and their gendered dimensions as 'dysfunctional communication' or 'poor parenting'.

The myth of the eating disorder family

The families of eating disordered women and girls have come in for much attention from medicine and psychology, and this has often involved blame and pathologisation through theories of abnormal development and dysfunctional family systems. However, to look at the role of the family in eating disorders does not have to mean adopting the developmental psychology so dominant in this area. As noted in previous chapters, abuse is situated in social contexts that are framed by gendered social relations (May-Chahal, 2006), and given that most physical, sexual and emotional abuse takes place within the family, these relationships are a key social site in which abusive relations are enacted in a day-to-day sense (Birrell and Freyd, 2006). As such, it is imperative to take a feminist sociological eye to girls' and women's experiences in families to better understand how abusive situations help to create such fertile conditions for eating disorders, as well as other common mental illnesses that are much more common in women.

Hilde Bruch's work in the 1960s and 1970s first posited the idea that the families of girls with anorexia shared certain features. Bruch (1978) suggested that these families were achievement-oriented, with mothers 'over-valuing' their anorexic child, or mothering 'too well' (Bruch, 1978). Anorexics were understood to have been deprived of independence, with the eating disorder a 'developmental crisis' (Bruch, 1978: 169) involving 'a desperate struggle for a self-respecting identity' (Bruch, 1974: 250). Research into family environments in eating disorders gained further ground in the 1970s with the emergence of family therapy and the idea of 'the anorexic family' (Palazzoli, 1974). Within this approach, communication patterns in the families of eating disordered individuals were assumed to be pathologically dysfunctional and enmeshed (Le Grange *et al.*, 2010). However, no such patterns were actually ever formally identified, and such assumptions resulted in widespread practices of family blame (Le Grange *et al.*, 2010). It is now generally acknowledged that many of the family dynamics observed in families where a member is struggling with an eating disorder are often in response to the eating disorder itself rather than necessarily reflective of pre-existing problems (Le Grange *et al.*, 2010). Nevertheless, the idea that the families of anorexic and bulimic women and girls are dysfunctional has held great sway for more than half a century and has contributed to the more general tendency to individualise eating disorders rather than consider wider social power relations and their realisation in day-to-day life.

While universalising assumptions about family pathology are very distressing for the many families where an eating disorder emerges in a caring and supportive environment, and they do, it is clear that abusive relationships substantially increase the risk. In exploring how women subjectively experience eating disorders in contexts of abuse, again, I am not concerned with establishing a linear causative relationship between the two. While physical, sexual and emotional abuse are widely reported (Arnow *et al.*, 2011; Finkelhor, 1994; Scher *et al.*, 2004; Scott, 2001) they do not necessarily result in eating disorders or other mental health problems for all individuals (Finkelhor and Berliner, 1995). As for other mental health problems, eating disorders are also understood to have multidimensional causes, involving socio-cultural, psychological, familial and biological aspects (Hund and Espelage, 2006; Streigel-Moore and Cachelin, 2001; Kent and Waller, 2000), with no one factor explanatory on its own. Although, as I also pointed out earlier, individual and family factors are usually given much more weight than social ones. Nonetheless, the one factor that stands above all others in the rise of eating disorders in Western and Westernising countries in the second half of the twentieth century is the cultural valuing of female thinness (Bordo, 2009), and it is within this wider social context that all other factors sit. Thus, what is of interest here is how women's subjective experiences of abusive family environments might frame subsequent experiences of an eating disorder in particular ways in socio-cultural contexts that value female thinness.

Abuse and eating disorders

Like all mental health problems that have been found to be more common among individuals with backgrounds of abuse, understandings of how abuse increases the risk of an eating disorder have been strongly influenced by psychological trauma models. In theorising eating disorders, trauma models suggest that any form of abuse involves boundary violations and a loss of trust resulting in low self-esteem, problems managing strong affect due to a diminished sense of self and general distress with an eating disorder understood as a 'maladaptive coping strategy' to manage these negative emotional states (Rorty and Yager, 1996; Hund and Espelage, 2006). Thus, abuse is understood as leading to problems with the regulation of emotion for which the eating disorder is the 'maladaptive' response (Rorty and Yager, 1996; Hund and Espelage, 2006). The idea that women with eating disorders have difficulty controlling emotion actually pre-dates the trauma model, though, and has been widely used to explain eating disorders more generally. Nevertheless, this is taken a step further in the trauma model where it is assumed that significant emotional trauma underlies difficulties in self-regulation and self-control for which anorexia and bulimia become the pathological, self-defeating solution.

While women who have experienced eating disorders and have histories of sexual abuse themselves link self-starvation and bingeing to the management of negative emotion, they actually describe quite specific feelings of guilt, self-hatred and powerlessness associated with childhood trauma, where the eating disorder is 'a powerful metaphor for or symbolic reliving of abusive experiences' (Rorty and Yager, 1996: 24). This hints at gendered social meanings and power relations in the emotional distress experienced by these women. However, such subjective interpretations and experiences are usually overlooked or dismissed within the psychological literature, including by the authors themselves in this case, on the basis that 'empirical research cannot, and need not, answer questions of individual meaning' (Rorty and Yager, 1996: 24). As noted in the previous chapter, this ignores the fact that subjective assessments of abuse are often of greater concern to individuals than the objective ones set down by researchers (Pelcovitz *et al.*, 1994) and are likely to be pivotal as to whether it is experienced as harmful or not (Downs and Miller, 1998). It also ignores the fact that individual meanings have a social dimension and do not simply emerge from the individual themselves. Clearly there are strong arguments for exploring at a more in-depth level individual experiences of eating disorders in contexts of abuse and the social dimensions of these.

Because eating disorders are mainly experienced by women (APA, 2013), they have also attracted much attention from feminist researchers and a substantial body of research now exists into their gendered dimensions (for example, Bordo, 2009; Malson, 1998). This has included critical interrogation of pathologising psychological discourses of eating disorders and the dysfunctional 'anorexic' or 'bulimic' family, particularly the once pervasive idea of inadequate mothering (Gremillion, 1992; Hepworth, 1999). While a small number of feminist scholars have also explored how sexual abuse plays a part in eating disorders for some women (Bordo, 1988, 2009; Wooley, 1994, 1996; Warin, 2010), as yet there has been no attention to other forms of abuse even though they are commonly experienced together (O'Hagan, 1993; Messman-Moore and Garrigus, 2007) and the impact appears to be greater when they are (Kent and Waller,

2000; Messman-Moore and Garrigus, 2007). The study presented here therefore represents the first attempt to explore through qualitative methods women's experiences of the development of an eating disorder in contexts of physical, emotional and sexual abuse.

Researching abuse and eating disorders

I undertook an in-depth interview study with 14 women who identified themselves as having experienced an eating disorder with the broader aim of exploring how they explain its emergence in their lives over time. As noted in the previous chapter, the study was not restricted to women as I was interested in differences according to gender, however, only women responded. While I expected abuse to emerge as a theme, I did not ask about it directly so as to allow participants to focus on the experiences they believed to be most relevant. Abuse was in fact one of the most common explanations for the emergence of an eating disorder in the women's lives. Again, the study was theoretically informed by McNay's (2004) concept of situated intersubjectivity, which understands the discursive aspects of identity and everyday material intersubjective power relations as intertwined (McNay, 2004). This is particularly unusual in feminist studies into eating disorders, which tend to be largely discursive. As with the other studies discussed in this book, I also brought a particular interest in the emotional dimensions of abuse and how these might play out in an eating disorder given the heavy emphasis on negative feeling as underpinning eating disorders in most of the literature. However, while psychological theories interiorise and pathologise emotion, as noted in Chapter 3, I drew on the post-structural feminist view of emotion as constituted in the intersubjective dynamics between individuals (Crawford *et al.*, 1992: 9) and as representative of 'the domain of the repressed that betrays the structure of regulation' (Burman *et al.*, 1996: 13) or the 'symbolic order' of repression (Weedon, 1987: 151). However, I also brought a materialist feminist understanding of emotion as lived in real bodies and as reflective of gender inequalities. As outlined in Chapter 3, a narrative-discursive interview method was used that unites attention to discourse and multiple identities with the more continuous aspects of lived narratives over time (Taylor and Littleton, 2006: 25) and their historical and social contexts (Riessman, 2008; Taylor and Littleton, 2006). Eating disorders usually emerge over many years so there are obviously continuous elements to the subjectivities involved.

The women participating in the study were aged between 19 and 49 years. They were recruited from the general community and a university campus via advertisements so that the sample was diverse in terms of type of eating disorder as well as class and cultural background of the women. This recognises that eating disorders are wider ranging than anorexia among white and more socially advantaged women, with bulimia and binge-eating disorders now the most common and all types experienced across class and racial groups (Bordo, 2009; Nasser and Malson, 2009; Sayers, 2009). Thus, seven of the women had experienced anorexia, three bulimia, two both anorexia and bulimia and two binge-eating disorder. Seven of the women identified themselves as coming from working-class or socially disadvantaged backgrounds, six identified middle-class backgrounds and one woman described a more socially privileged background. Lastly, three of the women were from non-English-speaking backgrounds including Middle-Eastern, Southern and Eastern European. A relatively unstructured approach to interviews was used so that women were given the opportunity to construct their narratives in the way they preferred, and I commenced by asking them to tell me about their lives and how they understood the place of an eating disorder within it. Many interviews became conversations when experiences were shared so the narratives are also to some extent co-constructions (Potter, 1996). The interviews ran for between one and two hours and were conducted either in my university office or in the women's homes depending on their preference. They were digitally recorded and transcribed verbatim.

Because this research involved a narrative-discursive analysis, the presentation of findings involves a mix of extracts to illustrate particular discourses as well as paraphrasing of key aspects of women's narratives to demonstrate the way experiences were linked and contextualised over time. Thus, as I am concerned with tracing the emergence of eating disorder symptoms in women's narratives over time, I have tried to keep their narratives relatively intact.

Abuse, food and the management of emotion

Nine of the women set their experiences of an eating disorder against a backdrop of emotional, sexual and/or physical abuse in their families of origin. Most of these women had experienced bulimia or binge-eating disorder, and although these numbers are small, this is nonetheless consistent with indications that these types of eating disorders may be most closely related to abuse (Deep *et al.*, 1999; Root and Fallon, 1989). Seven of the women disclosed sexual abuse, including repeated or one-off abuse by older males related or known to them, consistent with earliest reports of sexual abuse experiences among eating disordered women in the literature (Oppenheimer *et al.*, 1985), with varying levels of severity ranging from penetration to inappropriate touching (Fleming, 1997). Two women reported physical abuse involving repeated incidents of being hit by older family members such as parents or older brothers. Seven women described emotional abuse with some naming it as such and others describing experiences similar to Bernstein and Fink's (1998) definition outlined in Chapter 4. Most women had experienced both sexual and emotional abuse, and two of these had also experienced physical abuse. Three of the women not only mentioned childhood abuse but also emotional or sexual abuse from their partners in adulthood. Most women focused on the emotional impact of the abuse they experienced, particularly feelings of shame, guilt, sadness and self-loathing, and the role of the eating disorder in managing these. This is consistent with observations that it is emotion that drives the distress associated with abuse (Herman, 1997). While the women's narratives included a wide diversity of themes, they primarily situated their experiences of eating disorders as an emotional effect of abuse through three main thematic tropes:

1 self-nurturing through food;
2 self-punishment through food, and;
3 self-protection through food.

Pseudonyms have been allocated to the women to protect their identities.

Self-nurturing through food

Bingeing was portrayed in some women's narratives as a way of alleviating negative emotions emanating from abuse. Food is commonly associated with pleasure and comfort and this can be particularly so in less socially advantaged contexts where these may be in short supply in other life domains (Bordo, 2009). Connections between food and pleasure, home, comfort and safety are also often particularly strong in non-white cultures (Bordo, 2009). Three of the four women whose narratives described using food to reduce negative emotions from abuse came from either working-class or non-white backgrounds. They also specifically contrasted the pleasure and nurturance of food against the misery of abuse. Narratives offered by Rebecca, April, Carmel and Aisha are presented and analysed below, with particular attention to the socio-historical contexts surrounding the women's experiences of abuse and its emotional effects, and the specific ways these are portrayed as playing into bulimia and binge-eating disorder.

Rebecca is in her late forties and described her background as Celtic-Australian and middle-class. In tracing the emergence of bulimia in her late teens, Rebecca described early sexual abuse from her older brother and emotional abuse from her parents. She only learned of the sexual abuse as an adult, having no memory of it herself. As noted in the previous chapter, Rebecca talked about feeling frightened of physical intimacy by the time she reached adolescence and how adds here how she suspects the sexual abuse could be part of this:

> I was terrified of physical intimacy, right? Now, I think that comes from the fact that, and I've only just found this out recently … there was one little girl across the road [and I] used to pull down her pants and tickle her, and when I got to be about 12, I realised that what I was doing was really wrong, and so I stopped. And in counselling that I've had over the years, I've brought it up from time to time and they've always said, 'Well, who tickled you?' Right? So, then, I was talking to my older brother about this, maybe a couple of years ago he said, 'oh well, actually, that was me'. Because he was going to the scouts, and the scouts … would pin you down and tickle your genitals. So, it was a form of sexual abuse, really. And he was coming home and doing it to me, and I was only four and I don't know how long he'd been doing it to me.

N: And you didn't have a recollection of him doing it?

A: No, no. I was too young.

(Rebecca)

Having established this early experience as perhaps the original basis for her discomfort with her body, Rebecca went on to talk about becoming increasingly '*terrified*' about sex during puberty as described in the previous chapter in the extract where she was ordered to her room by her father because it was 'disgusting' that her brother should have to see her naked, developing body. Rebecca therefore identified powerful discourses about sex as 'dirty' and wrong, and about her female body as 'disgusting', as a further backdrop to growing shame and discomfort. In addition to this, Rebecca also described what she called 'emotionally abusive' treatment from her parents during adolescence and growing feelings of depression and low self-esteem over this period. In the previous chapter, Rebecca described being especially denied a voice and controlled through her parents taking the view that, as a girl, 'We have to mould you into who we want you to be because you've come from us', situating her as the property of her parents rather than an autonomous person in her own right. This offers a sociological understanding of the controlling family and the gender discourses and dynamics involved rather than a psychological one where controlling behaviour is simply a function of individual personalities and dysfunctional family dynamics. While Rebecca went on to mention being given other quite different messages to her brothers about marriage and dependency in addition to those surrounding sex and her body, she also described rebelling against these discriminatory expectations:

I was a rebel, I was a hippie, I had all these weird ideas, and it was like, 'Oh, why couldn't you be like so and so daughters?' So, I also developed this perfectionist thing because I was never good enough.... Once I became, when I sort of evolved into a young adult, let's say, 18, I had low self-esteem, I was very depressed, I had low self-confidence, I was really a mess, you know? My mum and dad had done a good job.

(Rebecca)

Rebecca therefore presented her rebellion against traditional values as the catalyst for further abuse and the subsequent development of low self-esteem and 'this perfectionist thing'. However, while Rebecca rebelled, she also wanted her parents' approval '*because I really loved them at some level, I really wanted to work it out with them*'. Thus, Rebecca positioned herself in the midst of a double-bind in wanting to develop her own identity but at the expense of parental love and support. While Rebecca's story could be understood as simply a personal account of abuse in an especially conflicted family, her narrative is framed by gender and class in quite specific ways. Hence, as a daughter, she experienced being denied autonomy and self-expression and felt particularly silenced and shamed about her body and sexuality as a girl. She also felt pressured to comply with a traditional, dependent femininity that reflected her parents' conservative, middle-class backgrounds but was out of step with 1970s Australia. This was a time when women were moving into the workforce and the feminist movement was active in making claims to gender equality and independence for women (Bulbeck, 1998). The so-called sexual revolution was also loosening sexual mores (Bulbeck, 1998). The abuse Rebecca described, and its structuring around highly conflicted expectations, is therefore framed by major shifts in gender discourses and relations in Western societies such as Australia at that time. There has been little attention to the psychological and emotional impact on women of the massive social changes of this period. While life opportunities undoubtedly widened, expectations about independence and sexual freedom did not simply supplant more traditional expectations in women's day-to-day lives but sat (and often continue to sit) alongside them in contradictory ways (Turner, 1992). Rebecca's narrative therefore captures a sharp disjuncture between what her parents expected of her and other ways of being on offer to young women at the time. The emotional consequences, as depicted by Rebecca, were that receiving love and support was conditional on performing a certain kind of femininity while failure to do so led to criticism and punishment and associated feelings of worthlessness, anxiety and sadness. Rebecca then went on to describe the specific situation in her late teens that initially triggered dieting:

R: I remember my older brother standing on the other side of the kitchen, and he looked at me and he said, 'Gee, you're fat'. Now, that was like the point where I started going, 'oh, I'm fat, I have to do something about this'. And, you know, when I look back, because there's so much in the media now, in relation to the tall and the skinny ... but you know, I think I must have been influenced ... because I remember feeling that if I wasn't thin, I wasn't attractive.

N: Ok, so there was a definite link?

R: There was a definite link. Yes, absolutely. And so I started starving myself, basically. And because I've always been a kind of person that really loves food, it was very hard. But I would starve myself for days and just pick on this, and pick on that, and I got pretty thin. I got down to a size 8, I think – 7½ [stone], and that was very thin for me, because I'm tall. And my periods stopped, but only for about four months. I was only actually anorexic for about a year before I discovered bulimia – binging and vomiting.

(Rebecca)

Rebecca therefore set her initial experiences of dieting within the wider conflation of female thinness with attractiveness. However, as her narrative progressed, it was the emotional impact of eating and not eating that became central rather than the pursuit of thinness per se. Rebecca said, '*I loved food and couldn't stand having this restricted life around food. I found that a complete bloody misery*'. It is not uncommon for bingeing and vomiting to start after women commence dieting to lose weight (Jacobi *et al.*, 2004), and Rebecca specifically emphasised the wretchedness of starvation and her realisation that food made her *'feel so much better about myself'*. Moreover, the shift from anorexia to bulimia was depicted as a conscious one when she said how she had *'discovered'* a way that she could eat without paying the price of weight gain. However, while food was presented as a panacea for feeling bad, it was also paid for with purging to prevent weight gain. Rebecca said, *'once I was like really bloated and faced with the task of having to go into that bathroom and throw it all up, I was like feeling like absolute shit, you know?'*. Thus, as is often the case for women, food is a guilty pleasure (Bordo, 2009; Hepworth, 1999), paid for with either purging or weight gain. In portraying the emotional roller-coaster of bulimia, Rebecca specifically drew on the explanation given to her by the psychiatrist she decided to consult when she felt the bingeing and purging were having too great an impact on her life:

> He went into the whole spiel about how it was a safety mechanism, and how the feelings of low self-esteem and low self-confidence, and the negative self-talk, which was really bad by this stage – 'you're a failure, you're never going to get anywhere, I hate myself' – it was really bad. And he said how this is like a safety mechanism where the binge eating is like, you go along, and you go along, and you take so much and it builds up, the emotional pain, the emotional pain, the emotional pain, and then you binge eat and you start to feel really good again. But then, after you binge eat it's like you're back where you started. And I thought, 'Yeah, this is right'.
>
> (Rebecca)

Rebecca described later walking out of treatment because this psychiatrist refused to acknowledge the role of abuse in her bulimia. However, here, she offered his cognitive-behavioural explanation of negative thoughts leading to escalating emotional distress that eventually culminates in bingeing to relieve these feelings. In common with cognitive-behavioural approaches more generally, negative thoughts are separate to and pre-exist relatively undifferentiated emotional distress (Briere and Runtz, 1993; Fairburn *et al.*, 1993). Splitting thought from feeling is universal within cognitivist psychology and has the effect of relegating emotion to the periphery in terms of its explanatory power as a disruptive and largely dumb force (Jaggar, 1989). As noted in Chapter 3, Williams' (1977) idea of structures of feeling re-theorises the relationship between thought and feeling as 'not feeling against thought, but thought as felt and feeling as thought' (Williams, 1977: 132). Thus, within this understanding, feeling is a social experience rather than a private and isolating one (Williams, 1977; Crawford *et al.*, 1992) with the emotions specifically meaningful rather than a single, totalising force (Gorton, 2007). Using this understanding, Rebecca's description of emotional pain can be understood as the shame, sadness and self-loathing that is part and parcel of thinking *'I hate myself'* and *'I am a failure'*. Furthermore, these feelings were specifically framed in her narrative by punishment for failure to meet the expectations of a more traditional femininity against other invitations to autonomy and self-expression. This is a quite different way of understanding the distress Rebecca described as not simply private difficulties in managing the trauma from abuse but as emotional conflict embedded in wider, historically specific gender discourses and practices. Thus, while psychological theories from this same period have historically portrayed eating disorders as a crisis of autonomy in girls in highly controlling parent–child relationships (Bruch, 1978), analysis of Rebecca's narrative demonstrates how what happens in families is historically specific, gendered and classed. As such, Rebecca's feelings of worthlessness, self-contempt and sadness become not simply personal troubles but reflective of wider contemporary social conflicts about expectations that women will be autonomous, independent and sexually assertive (living for themselves) and connected to others, caring and sexually passive (living for others) (see Turner, 1992), with the abuse Rebecca described structured around punishing the former and imposing the latter. Reconnecting thought with feeling in Rebecca's narrative therefore helps to illuminate the specific socio-historical and gendered nature of the emotions she described, with bingeing a way of trying to relieve these through the pleasure and nurturance of food. However, because food is a guilty pleasure for women, it also reproduces the shame and self-loathing so central to the vicious cycle of bingeing and purging.

April is in her early twenties and while her adolescence occurred some 30 years later than Rebecca's, there are nevertheless resonances in the way contradictory gender expectations are captured in the portrayal of her eating disorder, just as there were in Rose's, too, in the previous chapter. April described physical, sexual and emotional abuse as producing the emotional distress driving her bulimia. First, in a more extensive elaboration of an extract presented in the previous chapter, April spoke about the impact of physical and emotional abuse from her mother, a single parent struggling with serious mental illness:

> [My mother] was lying on the bed and struggling to breathe [during an asthma attack]. And then the day after when she recovered a bit, she blamed me and said that she could have died and it was my fault because I didn't help her, and she punched me. That was the first, the sort of beginning of it. It was the first time that my Mum ever hit me.... And also I started to sort of develop my own personality, like differentiate. So I started to like my music and wanted to choose my own clothes. And I think for my Mum that was really hard because I think she just wanted me to be like a little girl forever because she could control me. So, yeah, that was sort of the beginning of abuse.
>
> (April)

While this part of April's account echoes psychological discourses focusing on the role of controlling mothers in the development of eating disorders (Malson, 1998), her experiences of abuse were also set within an historical narrative of intergenerational physical, sexual and emotional abuse in her family:

My Mum is part Aboriginal and like, not Aboriginal by terms of culture, but just through skin colour, if you go on the basis of skin colour. And my brother is dark-skinned, and I know that she dislikes that part of herself as well. Because my Nanna was raped by an Aboriginal person, and then my Mum was born as a result of the rape. So my Nanna had a lot of mental health issues and was very abusive towards my Mum, and then she's done the same thing to my brother, and then after that was sort of me. Because I guess I'm a female and I resemble her in some way.... But since, well, actually before half of that stuff happened, she's also spent a lot of time in [a psychiatric hospital]. My Nanna spent a lot of time in [there] as well, while my Mum was growing up. And yeah, she's been diagnosed, like primarily with borderline personality disorder. And then I guess there's a secondary kind of diagnosis, narcissistic personality disorder, but the main one being borderline.

(April)

The abuse-related emotional distress in April's narrative is framed by gender in the way the effects of rape are specifically handed down intergenerationally from mother to daughter through rejection: hence, April said that as the only girl with two brothers, she was rejected and abused by her mother because '*I'm a female and I resemble her in some way*'. However, the abuse is also framed by race, with April asserting that her brother was emotionally abused because of his skin colour as her mother also '*dislikes that part of herself*'. April went on to say that once the abuse started, '*the biggest thing I had trouble with was emotionally.... I would just cry*' and that her mother's love and care '*was the biggest thing that I missed*'. April then described her experiences of sexual abuse by her older brother and how she came to realise at this same point in her life that '*it wasn't supposed to be happening*' when she received sex education at school:

A: And also at that stage, I had sex education, so I found out that a lot of things another person in my family was doing to me weren't supposed to be happening.
N: Was it in your family?
A: Yeah, so that was pretty shitty.
N: So that was one of the first times you could make any sort of meaning out of what had been happening as you learned that stuff at school?
A: Yeah. Because up until then I didn't really know any different. And that was when I first sort of turned to food as like a coping thing. And it wasn't until I was about 14 that I first started making myself vomit.
N: What motivated you to start vomiting?
A: I guess because I felt like I'd lost a lot of control and I was really worried about getting fat. And I compared myself to a lot of my friends who had really flat stomachs.

(April)

The way April described only becoming upset about her brother's behaviour when she learned that it was inappropriate highlights the significance of sub-jective meaning-making to the impact of child abuse (Downs and Miller, 1998). April almost never met my eye as she told me about the different types of abuse she had experienced, and while she did not directly name shame, she sat with her head downcast seemingly uncomfortable and ashamed (see Probyn, 2005). April moved on to talk about how she began '*turning to food and binge-eating as a way to comfort myself*' once the physical, emotional and sexual abuse started. She went on to describe the vicious cycle of bingeing and purging:

> It didn't last. The feeling of comfort only lasted as long as you were putting the food in your mouth and as soon as you stopped and you kind of realised what you'd done and the consequences of that, you felt even worse about yourself.
>
> (April)

In addition to at least temporarily relieving sadness from abuse, April also said that '*food doesn't argue back and food doesn't tell you what to do*', juxtaposing the power and pleasure of satisfying herself through bingeing against the feel-ings of powerlessness and sadness in abuse. In contrast to this, April portrayed purging as a way of controlling weight because '*I am really worried about getting fat, and I compare myself to a lot of my friends who have really flat stom-achs*'. Hence, as in Rebecca's narrative, the pleasure of food comes at a price and purging becomes a rational solution to the dilemma of needing the comfort of food while at the same time needing to remain thin. April also talked about the complicating problem of having Type 1 diabetes, and how the abdominal bloating caused by this leads to further distress about size and shape but also to avoiding insulin in order to lose weight, at great peril to her health and her life. April went on to say how she craves thinness and envies her friends:

> They're all like, it's probably just my perception, they're all really skinny and they're all beautiful and they all wear all the same sort of clothes and whatever. I find it so difficult when I'm with them. Like normally when I go out with them, I come home and I feel really depressed [with] the whole eating thing [and I say to myself] 'I'm not going to eat for a week'.
>
> (April)

April depicted her friends as successful, beautiful and thin and herself as aspir-ing to be like them, even though avoiding insulin and starving herself is risky to her health and deprives her of the comfort of food. Thus, April positioned herself in a continuing tussle with food, using bingeing to alleviate feelings of worth-lessness and sadness but then purging and starving to control weight. Similarly to Rebecca, in April's narrative, emotional abuse is framed by conflicted gender discourses and practices whereby she is punished for autonomous behaviour and expected to be '*like a little girl forever*' against efforts to assert her own identity and independence. Again, while psychological explanations of eating disorders identify a pubertal crisis of autonomy in the young woman herself (Crisp, 1980), as for Rebecca, April's narrative points to conflicted gender discourses and power relations that came into play during adolescence.

Carmel also emphasised the role of bingeing to alleviate emotional distress from abuse. She is in her late forties and identifies her background as working class. Carmel described experiencing emotional abuse from her parents during childhood and adolescence, and later from her husband. The abuse in her family of origin was mainly portrayed as emotional neglect, but she also described witnessing her father sexually assault her mother. In addition to these early experiences, Carmel gave particular emphasis to emotional abuse, neglect and financial abuse from her ex-husband both while they were married and after they divorced, and its impact on her sense of herself. She described ongoing financial problems as the context for financial abuse. She also portrayed a traditional arrangement in relation to gender roles, where she took responsibility the children and domestic chores as a stay-at-home mother, with her husband tightly controlling the finances and all decisions about spending:

> He wouldn't even hand money over to me, he'd just like give me money in the bank, like 'there's your money for the month', that was it. And it was very limited funds and I had to struggle. But as long as he could have his beer and time away.... As long as he had his money, he got his boat, he got, yeah, whenever, on his holidays and stuff.
>
> (Carmel)

Carmel also specifically referred to abuse about her weight from her ex-husband:

> He goes 'Oh if you lose weight I'll marry you now'.... I remember he said, 'Oh if you ever get fat I'll leave you'.... I just thought 'Did I just hear right?' And then I think my sub-conscious thought 'Stuff you, I'll eat' ... I don't know, maybe because he thought I come from gutter trash, he could treat me like gutter trash.
>
> (Carmel)

Carmel went on to say that '*basically my support system has been food*', however, her account also involved rebellion against her husband's threats of rejection through bingeing. In contrast to the contradictory gender expectations and discourses in Rebecca's and April's narratives, Carmel gave a more straightforward account of emotional abuse in a context of classed social disadvantage and traditional gender roles that positioned her with less power than her husband. In spite of indicating a rebellious aspect to bingeing, Carmel went on to primarily construct it as a product of low self-esteem and as a way of nurturing herself in this context:

> I just didn't feel worthy ... you just think 'oh what am I, chopped liver?' ... it just hurts because it makes you feel like you're invalid, like you've got no

self-worth and no self-esteem. And that's why I think I tolerated so much crap from [my husband] because I felt 'well, maybe I don't deserve any better'. And it's a trigger for eating, when I'm getting hurt ... so that's why I think, yeah, the food thing mattered to me.... It does feel nice when you're eating it. Because I used to buy a block of chocolate and I'd be like two pieces here, two pieces there, and before I know it, I've eaten the whole block and I'm like 'oh!' ... but then you feel really like you're such a fat pig, you know? And then you start feeling bad.... Yeah, it just feels nice at the time, it's like 'oh, I deserve this niceness, to have something nice going on'.

(Carmel)

As in the previous two narratives, the pleasure and comfort of bingeing is contrasted against the negative feelings of abuse, with food representing pleasure and self-nurturance in a context where these are otherwise in short supply. However, using food to self-nurture again came at a price when Carmel said how '*you feel really like you're such a fat pig*'. This is an evocative illustration of reconnecting thought with feeling and how this helps to elucidate the socio-historical context of emotional distress. Cognitivist psychological theory suggests one cannot *feel* fat: you can only *think* you are fat and, as a result, *perceive* yourself to be fat and then *feel* depressed and anxious. However, women often describe 'feeling fat' (Malson, 1998): it is possibly one of the best examples of a widely experienced structure of feeling among women in modern Western cultures obsessed with female thinness and self-control. In Carmel's narrative, then, while abuse-related feelings of worthlessness and shame are at least temporarily alleviated by bingeing, representing some '*niceness*' in her life, it also reinforces feelings of worthlessness, fatness and shame.

Aisha set her binge-eating disorder against the backdrop of a rape by a 60-year-old neighbour and its aftermath when she was 16. Now in her twenties, Aisha told me how she and her family came to Australia from the Middle-East as refugees ten years ago and how they had become friendly with their neighbour, who offered to give her a lift to school one day:

He was just my neighbour. He was living across the road. I missed the bus to go to school, and he offered to take me to school.... So, I accepted the offer, and I just whinged about – well I think, at that stage everybody hates school anyway, so I hated it. And then, he's like, well if you don't have to go to school – I don't have to drop you off at school if you don't want to. I said wow, really?... He actually just took me to [an isolated beach].... So, like at the beach, things just got funny and there was no one else on that beach. And the first thing that I told him, like just to take me back to – because I knew my parents – the first thing, like I just didn't want to get into trouble. So, he was like – well he wouldn't bring me back, and so, I told him, if he doesn't drop me off, like at three o'clock – that's the time that school would get out. So, if I didn't catch the same bus, or if my teachers haven't seen me, then they'll probably call my parents. So, it's better if he drops me off then.

N: So, you had to kind of bargain with him to get a way of getting back?
A: Yeah. Well I played it as if that I'm on his side, and that I want to do this, so that he would – because I had no idea where I was, so I thought, if I make him angry, he's um...

(Aisha)

While Aisha did not describe the rape in detail, she later mentioned having sustained a physical injury during it, suggesting that it was violent. Aisha said that she felt frightened by the rape itself but she gave most prominence to being blamed by her family later. As she said, '*I knew my parents*', and it is this experience that she set up as foreshadowing her subsequent struggles with binge-eating. In an elaboration of an extract presented in the previous chapter, Aisha described how she tried to prevent her parents learning of the rape because she knew she would be blamed:

I begged the school Principal not to [tell them about the rape] because, you know, in my culture it's, I don't know, they just, it's always your fault. I mean, they say, 'well you might have wanted it'. Because the problem was I was sixteen, I wasn't just like a five year old or someone who had no idea what's going on, and so I could have run, but I didn't. Or I could have screamed, but I didn't. So, that was the problem. So, my parents were quite mad at me for some time. For about a year, I couldn't get out of the house.

(Aisha)

As noted in the previous chapter, Aisha drew on a number of victim-blaming discourses and practices here including the idea that a dangerous female sexuality provokes rape; that women secretly want to be raped; and that that rape occurs because women fail to resist sufficiently (Gavey, 2005: 19). The gendered victim-blaming identified by Aisha therefore rests on highly contradictory discourses of female sexuality as passive and compliant *and* active and dangerous (MacSween, 1993: 178), with women positioned simultaneously as powerless sexual victims but at the same time responsible for predatory male sexual behaviour. Rather than directing anger towards her family, though, Aisha described feeling furious with the school principal for reporting the rape because she knew that she would be held responsible. Aisha's anger throws into relief the fact that this emotion was rarely mentioned or expressed by the other women in this or the previous reported study into childhood emotional abuse as a response to any form of abuse. This does not mean anger was not felt and more likely reflects continuing socio-cultural prohibitions surrounding its expression by women (Spelman, 1989). It also reflects the very real risks and social costs associated with expressing anger if the perpetrators of abuse are relatives or when relatives are holding a woman accountable for sexual assault or abuse, drawing attention to the complicating role of betrayal in violence against women (Gold-smith *et al.*, 2004). As noted in the previous chapter, Aisha went on to say how after being blamed for the rape, she '*couldn't get out of the house for a year*', and that her parents, primarily her father, '*just never trusted me again*'.

Aisha's narrative also included other complexities around gender and culture that serve as a backdrop to her construction of emotional distress from the rape and the development of binge-eating disorder. She mentioned that she has two older sisters but, to the great disappointment of her parents, no brothers. Aisha went on to describe how her father encouraged her until her mid-teens to take on the identity of the 'honorary son' and how she cut her hair short, wore boys' clothes and behaved differently to her sisters:

A: Well actually, I was supposed to be the son, and then, like yeah, but it didn't happen, so it disappointed everyone.... Until the age of 15 I wasn't allowed to grow my hair, and my Dad would always introduce me as his son. And if I wore boys' clothes I would get, like really, I mean, everybody would love it.

N: But you knew you weren't a boy?

A: I always thought I was a boy, but then you get to the stage where you have to decide – 'OK, I can't be a boy'.... I started growing my hair around – yeah when I was 16 – but I had lots of arguments with my Dad.... I mean, the whole family didn't like it. They were just used to me being the boy of the family. Because I mean, I would always to what guys normally do. I would try to fix the car, and yeah.

N: So, you really took on this role, like you were behaving quite differently to your two sisters in the family?

A: Yeah, because that was the only way that [my parents] would get close.

(April)

This account challenges assumptions about gender roles in cultures where they are assumed to be quite fixed, but it also portrays the receipt of love and approval as wholly conditional on performing a masculine identity. Moreover, while the adoption of a feminine identity was presented as bringing disapproval and emo-tional distance, it later brings punishment, blame and rejection in the context of rape. Having talked about the events surrounding the rape, Aisha went on to describe problems with binge-eating and the persistent insomnia that developed afterwards:

But after everything, I had problems with sleeping. And so, I would be awake the whole night. So, I thought, if I just eat.... So, it did work but it still, I don't know.... It's not the food, I think I'm more worried about not being able to go back to sleep.... But obviously, when I'm going to have something, I'll have something nice ... so I've gained a lot of weight.... I've tried to stop it but it hasn't happened.... Sometimes I kind of don't open my eyes because I'm tired. But I don't really look at the amount. Or sometimes, I don't even remember how much I ate, I'll wake up the next day and I'm like, 'Oh, wow, what have I done again?'. But I don't know, if I don't eat, then yeah, I get really scared that I won't be able to sleep.

(Aisha)

Aisha described feeling anxious about her night-time bingeing and subsequent weight gain but she was also confused about how, or even if, it relates to the rape. Being blamed is known to complicate the effects of sexual assault for women (Levett, 2003), and insomnia is a well-known reaction to the trauma of rape and sexual abuse (Herman, 1997). However, Aisha found it difficult to identify or talk about her feelings in response to these experiences. She described instead envying other young people whose mothers seem to provide unconditional support and care for them, and avoiding seeking professional help for fear of further rejection and becoming dependent on support: she said, *'that's what I'm worried about, what if I do want the support all the time?'* Instead, she is the carer of her mentally ill mother and remains estranged from her father. Aisha's narrative is therefore intersected by gender and culture in particularly complex ways and the fear, anger, rejection, isolation and longing for support that she described, and its relationship to insomnia and binge-eating, cannot be well-understood without reference to this multifaceted context.

In each of the four narratives above, gendered experiences of emotional, sexual and physical abuse drive the emotional distress underpinning bulimia and binge-eating. Here, food holds contradictory meanings and functions as both nurturing and prohibited, with bingeing providing pleasure and relief from emotional distress but also self-censure and pain because of the risk of weight gain and further social rejection. In marked contrast to the construction of self-nurturing through food, two other women described using food to punish themselves in contexts of abuse.

Self-punishment through food

Both Louise and Carole focused on the use of food as self-punishment for abuse, particularly for sexual abuse. Louise is in her mid-twenties and described her background as relatively privileged. As noted in the previous chapter, she talked about physical, emotional and sexual abuse having led to dissociative identity disorder and anorexia nervosa:

Growing up I was basically sexually abused for most of my childhood.... But then there was a lot of physical violence in the home, there was a lot of manipulation [by my father, so] by the time I was fifteen I was hearing voices, self-harming a lot ... and then by the time I was twenty-ish, I was diagnosed with dissociative identity disorder.

(Louise)

Louise mentioned extreme sexual abuse at the hands of her father and his friends that continued for many years. I was very cognisant of the fact that she seemed reticent to disclose details of the abuse so, as advised by Warner (2009), I did not press her and focused instead on its effects. Louise told me that when she began experiencing extreme dissociation in adolescence, including the presentation of alternate personalities, self-harming and severe anorexia, not one adult in her life connected this with the possibility of sexual and other forms of childhood abuse. As an example, she described writing a story at school about the abuse:

> I'd done, in year 12, it was a creative writing piece basically, and you go through and the whole story, basically about how shit my life is and it's talking about someone's rage and you know, being abused and everything, and then you get to the last line, oh, and it talks about I want to die, and then the last line is basically that I can't because I'm a rock on the beach, and my abuser is the ocean, and my [new] doctor just read it and she just went 'How could nothing have been reported about that' like she said … there's so much a culture of, you don't want to know … the principal saw it, and everyone saw it, and I look back now and I'm like, 'why did no one say anything?'
>
> (Louise)

Warner (2009) points out that professionals do not always want to know about sexual abuse and can therefore avoid raising it, particularly if an individual is seen to be vulnerable. As noted earlier, Louise was at pains to emphasise that emotional and physical abuse were also relevant to her mental health problems because it is so easy to dismiss in the face of such extreme sexual abuse:

> But then, I would say kind of, on top of that, there's a lot of, like there was physical violence in the home, there was, a lot of, manipulation, like, a lot of games going on, so, it was kind of … a lot of, one minute you know that you're fantastic and you know you can't do anything wrong, and that you're loved, and then the next minute it's, you're a selfish bitch for asking for help and just never knowing where you stand. So it's that kind of, everything can seem perfect one minute, but, when it blows up it really blows up, and kind of, you know, one minute you're getting the best grades, and you know, you're great, you work hard, and you deserve it, and then it's, no, no, no, it's because you're not working hard enough that you, and so it's just that never knowing.
>
> (Louise)

Building on Louise's account of mixed messages offered in the emotional abuse study, here she depicted physical and emotional abuse as revolving around conflicted messages about identity and worth so that she found herself swinging between 'perfect daughter' and 'selfish bitch'. The emphasis on academic achievement mentioned here is also highly gendered and classed because achieving at school is particularly expected of girls (Walkerdine *et al.*, 2001) and is the most powerful form of cultural capital for the middle classes (Reay, 1997): only those women in the wider study identifying as middle or upper class talked about family pressure regarding academic performance in the development of their eating disorders. Louise was also one of only two women disclosing abuse who struggled exclusively with anorexia rather than bingeing and purging, and next she talked about how feelings of unworthiness and self-contempt related to abuse played into self-punishing starvation:

> There's a strong connection to self-harm, there's a lot of stuff around 'I don't deserve to eat this', kind of like self-hate ... there was times when I was really unwell, where I wouldn't eat, but, you know, I wouldn't let myself sleep in a bed, because I wasn't worthy of sleeping in a bed, I'd sleep on the floor.
>
> (Louise)

Here, starvation and the discomfort of sleeping on the floor are punishments driven by abuse-related feelings of self-hatred and unworthiness. However, these practices also suggest penance and atonement, which in turn suggest feelings of culpability and guilt (Levett, 2003). Using self-starvation as a form of self-punishment and atonement has been previously identified by Malson (1998) in the narratives of women with anorexia, but connections with feelings of shame and guilt related to sexual abuse, and other forms of abuse too, have not been previously drawn. This adds a powerful and more profoundly gendered dimension to practices of self-starvation in the context of sexual abuse. Next, Louise went on to specifically explain how anorexia emerged in the context of abuse-related DID:

> With dissociative identity disorder, like you lose time, so I'd have big components of time that I just don't remember stuff, and obviously like the abuse stuff, because it's never really been dealt with, like it's being dealt with now, but, you know.... I had no control over my situation because I couldn't tell the family what was going on, they were just like, 'hey my daughters a fuck up and I don't know why', like, so ... It felt like basically my life was completely out of control, and, I remember quite clearly sitting in an emergency room once, when, you know, they're basically saying, you know, 'you're too underweight you're going to have be admitted' kind of thing, and they were talking about what's going on, and I said, 'well I can't control anything in my life, but I can control what goes into my mouth, and I can control my weight, and you know, if I can be perfect by being skinny, then, you know, that's something, like I may be failing in every other aspect of my life, but my weight I can control, and that's me, and me only.... I may not be good enough at anything else, in anyone else's standards, but, you know, if I'm skinny, I'm showing to the world that I can, that I am perfect in something', so.
>
> (Louise)

In this extract, anorexia is a remedy for an extreme sense of lack of control wrought by the symptoms of DID and the need to hide severe sexual abuse from the world, providing Louise with a way of '*showing to the world that I can, that I am perfect in something*'. Louise went on to explain further how thinness became a '*mask*' or '*disguise*' to the outside world for abuse and DID:

> I've often talked about anorexia being my disguise, like it's, kind of like a mask to the outside world of, what's really going on, it's, I don't know … For me it hides everything else that's going on, like, all the hallucinations, the, not having control over so much and feeling so out of control, that if to the world I can portray an image that I am in control, and that everything's good, then, you know, then it is, it's a disguise, and it's a disguise that it does throw people off, like, when you are, you know, 40, 45kg or whatever, people don't focus on what else is going on … because they are, they're more focused on, you know, is this person picking up their fork to eat, or are they, you know, going to the bathroom straight after a meal.
>
> (Louise)

Thus, Louise presented the thinness of anorexia as both a means of hiding abuse but also as a way to overcome the shame and guilt associated with it: as suggested by Bordo (2009), anorexia in such contexts can be understood as 'a fantasy of control and invulnerability, and immunity from pain and hurt' (Bordo, 2009: 52). At the time of interview, Louise's experiences of sexual abuse had not been disclosed to her family. She volunteered for a second interview in the childhood emotional abuse study two years later and with the support of her new psychiatrist, the sexual abuse had been disclosed to her family by that stage and while not fully acknowledged, both her dissociative symptoms and anorexia were improving significantly.

In contrast to Louise's focus on self-starvation as punishment for sexual, emotional and physical abuse and a mask for emotional distress, Carole set her bulimia against the back drop of blame for a rape perpetrated by her ex-husband following their separation. However, she first described a history of gendered and classed family and partner abuse that she believes set her up to feel that she 'deserved bad treatment'.

> I was raised in … a quite a rough part of the country. I've got four older brothers. I'm the youngest of five. I had a pretty interesting childhood with my parents, a very disruptive sort of childhood. My parents finally, after many years, divorced when I was about 15.… My Dad went to prison when I was two, so mum was on her own with the five of us.… And then [after he got out], my dad was very much what they would call a man's man, and he was out drinking.… And Mum was at home and obviously, very resentful. And the way she dealt with it was through alcohol and valium, and taking it out on the kids, being very – she had a lot of issues herself but she was very dramatic,

real attention seeking. She went for a period over a couple of years of just taking overdoses, trying to kill herself, so it really affected all of the kids, obviously. My older two brothers were, like nine and ten years older, so them not so much, and they just basically, moved away because they didn't want to have anything to do with it.... But the other two sort of moved out when they were around 14 and 15 years of age ... so then, it was left to me. I was pretty much stuck with being the carer of my mum from very young. Yeah, a couple of times I was on my own with her when she was attempting to kill herself, around about 12.

(Carole)

Carole therefore described a conflict-ridden childhood and adolescence in a disadvantaged family where, as noted in the previous chapter, she was left with the responsibility of caring for her mentally ill mother as the only daughter with four brothers. She then talked about marrying young in part to escape, and experiencing further emotional neglect from her first husband:

I'd put up with a lot of bad behaviour. He was a gambler and whatever, and very neglectful, affectionately, very neglectful, but I put up with that.... It was neglectful emotionally ... he would gamble the money, and took no responsibility for that action at all, just a very, very selfish person. But then, I'd been brought up with very selfish people and thought that that was the kind of treatment that you should accept, because I didn't know any different and I didn't know people ... that you didn't deserve that.

(Carole)

As noted, Carole saw the abuse she experienced in childhood as setting her up to accept later intimate partner abuse, going on to say '*I didn't know any better sort of thing ... you have this – that you deserve it, you know?*' Next, Carole moved on to specifically explain how her bulimia was triggered. She described separating from her former husband and then discovering shortly afterwards that she was pregnant to him. Carole chose to terminate the pregnancy and her ex-husband raped her when he learned about this:

C: This was probably a day or two after I'd had the termination, and he raped me, because he wanted to put that child back.... I was really, obviously not in a good head space.... But after a few weeks I couldn't get it out of my head, it felt like it was some kind of dirty secret that only he and I knew about. So, I did report it. And the police knew that I was telling the truth, they knew. And the officer, you know, I'll always be very grateful because he was ... (too upset to talk).

N: Oh look, do you want to stop for a minute?

C: No, no, no.

N: Are you sure?

C: It isn't the, it isn't the actual.... It isn't the actual act of what he done that actually upsets me, it's actually the kindness of the officer that – emotion affects me – ridiculous, and I don't know why.

N: No it's not, I think that's really understandable.

C: Yes it's strange, he was – he said, and because naturally, you think that they're not going to believe you. You just think, people are not going to believe you. But he knew.... So, after that I basically collapsed really. I think I became very, very unwell – mentally, very unwell, and just really wanted to turn to suicide. So, it was my sort of, every thought of how I could do it, when I would do it, how it would affect the kids, because I still had this immense love and responsibility towards my children, and that was really, sort of pulling me that you can't do that, because what that then, you're being as selfish as your mother was, and I didn't want to put that on my children. And I basically, couldn't do it, I couldn't allow myself to be selfish enough to take my life.

N: So, that's what pulled you back?

C: And that is – I think, I can actually remember very distinctly lying in bed and being very conscious of breathing, and really, it was as if a part of me was actually looking at me. It felt as if myself had come out.

N: You were outside looking in?

C: Yeah looking in at me, and basically, saying 'you are, you're going to either die, or you've got to get better'.... It was almost amazing, yeah really, so peculiar that insight, you know?

(Carole)

Carole portrayed the rape as an act of revenge by her ex-husband for having had a termination of pregnancy and a way of reclaiming ownership over her body by seeking to '*put that child back*'. As is pointed out by Warner (2009), men who perpetrate sexual assault often intend for the woman to feel she deserved it. Carole also described expecting not to be believed, and her surprise and gratitude when the police officer accepted the veracity of her report. Lastly, she described feelings of love and responsibility for her children as preventing her from committing suicide. Part of this included a description of dissociation, where Carole experienced herself as outside her body and therefore removed from distress (Herman, 1997). This is a common response to trauma, including sexual assault (Herman, 1997), and here Carole presented it as instrumental in choosing to live and recover. She also went on to specifically describe how she moved from a dissociative suicidal state to bingeing and purging, and the role of self-blame in this:

C: And so, I pulled myself together, but from that developed some OCD [obsessive compulsive disorder] with constant washing myself, and bathing, and in Dettol and trying to clean myself.... It was awful. I wanted to have all my womb taken out. I wanted to try and, I would imagine cutting it out with a knife, myself. I wanted to cut my breasts off, because there I was thinking, well I caused this because I'm female, that it was my fault because I was a female. Rather than putting that blame with that person and saying, actually it wasn't my fault, it was my fault because he either found me attractive, so I was too attractive, so what can I now do.

N: As if somehow it was something about you?

C: Yeah, so, I then developed an eating disorder.

(Carole)

Carole presented the sexuality of her body as having effectively caused the rape (Gavey, 2005) so that the desire to strip it of its female sexual characteristics becomes protective as well as punitive and driven by self-loathing. In explaining the bulimia further, she was adamant that '*it wasn't about being slim. I didn't want to be slim, I didn't want to be attractive*', rather '*the voice in my head was telling me that I deserved it*'. She said:

C: I would binge for hours, but I would actually be cramming the food in to hurt myself.

N: So it was like a punishment sort of thing?

C: It was a punishment, yes.... And the food that I would eat, it was revolting, because I didn't have money to buy nice food. It would be anything that you could put together ... and just ram, ram, ram. And then, after that the shame and the feeling so guilty for what I'd done. And then, all of that hurt and punishment I'd just stuffed into me I now needed to get out of me, because I didn't really deserve it, so then ... the purge would take place, and then I'd take laxatives, and then I would be in the bath, scrubbing myself because I'd done that, and because of the sexual abuse, and I was just really caught up in this really horrible cycle.... And nobody knew, nobody knew.

(Carole)

Bingeing offered protection from further sexual assault, indicated in Carole's insistence that she didn't want to be slim or attractive (Root and Fallon, 1989). More than this, though, she described swinging between secretive self-punishing binges and self-purifying purges with her body the object of hate – '*ram, ram, ram*' – in a seeming re-enactment of the dynamics of the rape itself, leaving her feeling guilty and ashamed. Connections between forced sex, forced food and disgust are apparent (also see Warin, 2010), with Carole particularly describing the food as '*revolting*' because it was cheap. Here, food and bingeing become a weapon rather than a pleasure in a parody of the way forced sex is a weapon in rape (Herman, 1997), with purging and scrubbing an attempt to cleanse away the defilement of both. Moreover, Carole took the blame because, as she said earlier with disconcerting simplicity, '*it was my fault because I am female*'. However, she also experienced swinging between positions of fault and innocence because, at another level and symbolised in the expulsion of guilt through purging, she said '*I now needed to get [it] out of me, because I didn't really deserve it'*. Again, conflict is central to this experience, with bingeing and purging the respective embodiments of this.

Re-enacting sexual abuse through self-harming starvation, bingeing and purging has been widely identified in the psychological literature (for example, Rorty and Yager, 1996). However, rather than understanding this as pathological and an end in and of itself, the self-punishment depicted by Louise and Carole involved an attempt to overcome the distress of abuse through purposeful rituals of punishment, restitution and absolution from guilt and shame based on symbolic connections between food, eating and sex. The connection with Christian rituals of confession, penance and absolution are clear and other authors have observed that anorexia in particular often involves aesthetic and self-punitive practices with strong religious overtones (Bell, 1985; Malson, 1998; Bordo, 1988). However, what is also apparent here is the profoundly gendered nature of self-blame and self-punishment in the context of sexual abuse and rape, as well as physical and emotional abuse. In addition to self-punishment, Louise and Carole also referred to the idea of self-protection from further sexual abuse through starvation and bingeing, and this idea is examined in greater detail through analysis of Helena's narrative.

Self-protection through food

In Louise's account, starvation and the mask of anorexia were presented as an invulnerable front to the world, while Carole sought a level of self-protection through bingeing based on the idea of not wanting to be thin and therefore attractive to men. In Helena's narrative, self-protection and the management of sexual attention from men emerged as the main function of her anorexia in the context of sexual abuse. Helena is in her late forties and described her background as middle-class and second-generation Eastern-European. She set her anorexia against a background of sexual abuse at the hands of the father of one of her friends at 12 years of age, and then later from two much older male cousins. In the following extract, one of a number of instances, she not only emphasised her fear during the assault itself but, like Aisha, being blamed later:

H: He was like a family sort of friend but also my brother's godfather. I went to a BBQ and we were running around and I was just wearing jeans and a halter-neck top, you know, the seventies fashion and basically it was just normal kids clothing, you know, because you're only 12 ... and for some reason he grabbed me and I was developing so I was curvy. You know, I was probably a size 10–12, curvy but very similar height to what I am now ... but it was a dark area and it was outside and he just grabbed me in the bushes and just stuck his hands down my top and he just held them there for a long time but it seemed like an eternity. And I just couldn't say anything, I was just terrified, I couldn't scream, I couldn't do anything.

N: Like you were almost sort of frozen?

H: Yeah, I was just terrified, because no one had ever done that before and it was just, it seemed like I was obviously assaulted. I didn't even understand it. Because I'd only just really found out the facts of life, you know, pretty much. I'd only just got my period like a short time before and my cousin had explained the facts of life to me because my Mum never did and it only just, like I was just pretty innocent. And anyway, then he let me go, but it just seemed like a long time, and then we were inside and I think I tried to tell my Mum and she'd been drinking ... she just said 'oh well, you shouldn't have been wearing that top, it wasn't appropriate' or something. She sort of put it down to that.

N: Put it back on you basically?

H: Yeah, basically, yeah. It made me feel uncomfortable. And so yeah, that sort of probably left an impact and then later that night we were sitting there and he had this sleazy look on his face and he said 'oh, I'm sorry about what happened'.

(Helena)

Helena tells me this with a level of incredulity that she was held responsible for a sexual assault at such a young age and not her adult male attacker, going on to emphasise that while she was '*curvy*' at 12, she was '*pretty innocent*' and her style of dress was '*just normal kids clothing, you know?*', in an effort to counter blame all these years later. While the discourses surrounding sexual assault may be less overtly victim-blaming now than they were some 35 years ago when this took place (Gavey, 2005; Gavey and Schmidt, 2011), the idea that a woman's behaviour and dress means she is 'asking for it' still persists and assumes men cannot control their sexual urges and that women are responsible for gatekeeping this (McMahon, 2007: 365). Helena goes on to describe memories of her cousin, who was some ten years older, behaving inappropriately towards her:

He seemed to be in my room, in the shower, everywhere, but I don't think we actually had intimacy, I don't remember. And always with my body, but I can't remember anything really. And he was kissing me and I think he thought he was my [boyfriend], and he said if I wasn't his cousin, how this and this and this would've happened. But because I was so innocent and hadn't had any experience it was sort of like all over my head.

(Helena)

In a further instance, another much older cousin convinced Helena to undress and took photos of her and, once again, she was held responsible, this time by her aunt's family. She said '*he had initiated it, because I wouldn't have thought about taking my clothes off*'. Like Rebecca, Helena also described feeling '*uncomfortable*' about her changing body in puberty because of the reactions of those around her:

I remember during puberty, [my mother] came in my bedroom and I was undressed ... and she was saying 'oh, I think you better put some clothes on, because you don't want anyone else to see you like that', and it made me sort of a bit self-conscious but I had just started developing and maybe she was worried that, you know, I don't know, people coming onto me or whatever, I don't know what she was concerned about. But she made me sort of feel a bit self-conscious about my own body.

(Helena)

Helena went on to say how '*I was messed up emotionally with all this stuff going on*' and while she did not name shame explicitly, she implied it when she mentioned feeling uncomfortable and self-conscious about her body. After outlining her experiences of sexual abuse during adolescence and her increasingly mixed feelings about her body, Helena's narrative then moved in a fairly unstructured way through experiences of self-starvation and over-exercising followed by attempts to eat more and gain weight. She dated extreme dieting and over-exercise to the accident of having been fitted with braces during adolescence and losing weight as a result of not being able to eat because of the pain, for which she received many compliments from friends and family, drawing her attention to the social value placed on female thinness. She went on to refer over and over to her '*curvy shape*', its fluctuations according to her weight and her ambivalent feelings about it. For example, she said:

H: I actually had a real curvy shape from [starting to eat more]. And guys, you know, did find me attractive, but because I didn't have any boundaries, I did have some intimate times with guys but again, that probably shouldn't have happened because I wasn't in love, but it was just, I didn't really have the boundaries.
N: So they would be coming on to you?
H: They would be coming on to me and I didn't know what to do. So I just sort of basically sometimes just would put up with it because of what had happened with my cousin.

(Helena)

In Helena's narrative, weight gain was very often linked to her '*curvy shape*' and attention from men, experienced as both flattering but also out of control and frightening in that she sometimes felt unable to refuse the pressure to have sex with them. Thus, sex was '*something I would just put up with*' and she specifically drew on a psychological discourse about connections between histories of abuse and deficient personality boundaries in making this point (Rorty and Yager, 1996). While the links between sexual abuse and the eating disorder are more difficult to track in Helena's narrative, she described highly ambivalent feelings about her body as a desired object but also the catalyst for sexual abuse and harassment for which she is positioned as at least partially responsible through her appearance and her inability to refuse sex. Further to this, controlling weight in Helena's narratives seemed related to controlling sexual attention from men in the absence of other means of power and control in heterosexual encounters. Changes in weight have been previously identified as a means by which women sometimes seek to protect themselves from further sexual abuse (Warner, 2009). The only other method of refusal that Helena felt open to her was to ignore men who made unwanted advances:

> H: If a guy liked me and then I didn't feel comfortable, I'd just basically ignore them.
> N: So that was the way to sort of manage it?
> A: Yeah, just totally ignore them.

(Helena)

While Helena put her inability to refuse sex down to 'boundary problems', thereby placing blame on herself, saying 'no' to sex is commonly experienced by women as extremely difficult in the context of the unequal gender power relations surrounding heterosexual sex and the absence of a language that enables women to comfortably refuse (Gavey, 2005). It is not so difficult to see how such conditions might be keenly felt by women who have been shamed, blamed and silenced through previous sexual abuse, and how the control of body weight might be linked to managing this in a social context that places great value on female thinness and self-control but, at the same time, offers women limited scope for exercising power in heterosexual relations.

Gendered abuse, emotion and eating disorders

While previous feminist research has emphasised the gendered nature of childhood sexual abuse (Warner, 2009), analysis of these narratives as well as those in the previous chapter illustrates the different ways that childhood emotional and physical abuse can also be highly gendered. Moreover, the narratives demonstrate how multiple forms of gendered abuse can work to reinforce and compound its emotional impact, with some women describing how early emotional abuse set them up to feel they deserved later sexual assault and intimate partner abuse. More specifically, as in the previous chapter, the abuse depicted in most women's narratives rested on highly conflicted discourses and expectations about gender. Hence, some women described emotional and physical abuse focused on expectations they would be non-sexual, dependent and care for others against more contemporary invitations to autonomy and independence while sexual abuse involved a contradictory positioning as both passive victim and as responsible for abuse. As has been previously argued, within a post-structural feminist understanding, subjectivity is the site of conflicting and competing subject positions where emotional conflict arises when individuals attempt to 'reconcile the irreconcilable' in 'the attempt to take up a single, unified position in competing or incoherent discourses' (Weedon, 1987: 150). Eating disorders have been theorised as a particularly evocative illustration of an attempt to reconcile the irreconcilable. Bordo (1990) argues that the contemporary prefer-ence for female thinness that underpins the rise in eating disorders in consumer societies is traceable to disruption and change in traditional gender relations dating from the 1960s and reflects fear of, and a need to contain, a dangerous female desire that threatens male power. On the other hand, she also argues that thinness is attractive to and pursued by women themselves because it represents liberation from a domestic, maternal femininity and an embrace of 'male' coded qualities of autonomy, detachment and control that are highly valued in phallo-centric cultures (Bordo, 1990). While the pursuit of thinness itself was not always explicit or in the foreground of the women's narratives, similarly con-flicted ideas about femininity as living for others versus living for oneself struc-tured the women's experiences of abuse and were reflected in their subsequent struggles over food and weight. Thus, cultural ambivalences about femininity do not only operate at an abstract or distant level in media images of thinness: they also play out in women's day-to-day lives in micro-level intersubjective power relations that may appear to have little to do in any direct sense with food and weight per se but nevertheless become caught up with them in a culture preoccu-pied with female thinness and self-control. More specifically, gendered forms of abuse in many of these narratives not only reflected, but magnified, wider cul-tural ambivalences about femininity, producing powerful emotions that played out in the use of food as a similarly conflicted solution because, for women, it involves both pleasure and pain. However, while conflicted gender discourses were identified in most of the narratives, they were not apparent every account. Carmel in particular set her binge-eating disorder and abuse-related feelings of shame and worthlessness within a more uni-dimensional gendered and classed frame of partner abuse, traditional gender roles and social disadvantage. However, this account shared with most of the others a centring of shame as the pivotal emotion driving the eating problem.

While a variety of emotions were mentioned by the women in response to abuse, most particularly referred or alluded to shame and the closely related feelings of worthlessness, guilt, self-contempt and self-blame, with references to these sometimes indirect because of the shaming effects of naming shame (Probyn, 2005). As noted in the previous chapter, research has linked child-hood abuse with shame (Hoglund and Nicholas, 1995). Loader (1998) sug-gests that 'child abuse is all about shame ... the family curse of child abuse is the curse of shame' (Loader, 1998: 53). While this probably overstates the case because other emotions are also important (Budden, 2009), it neverthe-less draws attention to the centrality of shame to abuse and related feelings of guilt and self-loathing. Most importantly, though, shame is gendered (Probyn, 2005) and this is not well-understood within psychological theorisations. As shown, the women described being shamed about their developing bodies, sexualities and weight, and others about their fledgling attempts to assert themselves and forge their own identities as young women against more tradi-tional gender expectations of dependence, deference and caring for others. The gendered nature of shame and shaming was particularly obvious in the women's experiences of sexual abuse, with Carole's and Louise's explanations of using food to punish themselves powerfully demonstrating how ritualistic, punitive and purifying forms of both anorexia and bulimia can be tied to gendered discourses and practices that blame and shame women and girls for sexual abuse. In her analysis of shame, Probyn (2005) outlines Lehtinen's (1998) argument that shame for women is located in the cultural phenomenon of 'women's enduring, historically diverse, and multi-dimensional experiences of subordination' (Lehtinen, 1998: 68, cited in Probyn, 2005: 83). Thus, women most likely feel shame as more penetrating and internal than men do (Lehtinen, 1998, cited in Probyn, 2005: 83), while those who have experienced early and repeated shaming are likely to have an increased capacity to re-experience it later (Probyn, 2005). It is not so difficult to see, then, how the shaming of girls and women through gendered emotional, sexual and physical abuse might be reactivated in diverse and complex ways around food, eating and body weight in cultures that reify female thinness and self-discipline, and scorn female fat and self-indulgence.

While shame is undeniably a distressing and uncomfortable emotion, Probyn (2005) also draws on Silvan Tomkins' idea that shame is productive because it 'operates only after interest or enjoyment has been activated' (Sedgwick and Frank, 1995: 5, cited in Probyn, 2005: ix). Thus, we cannot feel shame about things we do not care about (Probyn, 2005). Probyn (2005) suggests that this interest 'describes a kind of affective investment we have in others' and is therefore about the desire for connection and reciprocity, and fear of contempt and abandonment (Probyn, 2005: 13). The shame of abuse can be seen as particularly powerful and distressing because the lost reciprocity and connection is with people with whom this was once shared, that is, family, friends and partners, and therefore involves significant levels of betrayal (Freyd, 1997). Some of the women alluded to the depth of this betrayal and loss when they described their yearning for reconnection with their families. Thus, as Rebecca said of her relationship with her parents '*I really loved them on some level, I really wanted to work it out with them*', while April said how emotional support from her mother '*was the biggest thing that I missed*' after the abuse started and Aisha yearned for the support and care of her mother after the rape. Moreover, most of the women placed more emphasis on being blamed and shamed for sexual abuse and rape by people close to them than the distressing experience of the assaults themselves.

In the women's narratives, then, one of the main functions of self-starvation and bingeing was to relieve gendered feelings of shame, worthlessness, rejection, sadness, anger, fear and self-loathing associated with such a fundamental abandonment and loss of connection. This contrasts with psychological notions of abused individuals needing to relive trauma in a psychopathologically compulsive way because it emphasises instead their efforts to *overcome* it through these practices (Herman, 1997). Thus, for some, self-nurturance or self-punishment through food offered a sense of reconnection with self and others while, for others, the social acceptance and connection that thinness seemed to promise was understandably appealing in the context of severe rejection. But self-starvation and bingeing could also function as a means of self-protection against further sexual abuse in the absence of other avenues of power in hetero-sexual relationships. Moreover, as noted, for most of the women, feelings of shame and worthlessness arose in social contexts characterised by profound ambivalence, with highly conflicted gender expectations and conditional rela-tionships providing fertile ground for shaming across various dimensions of their lives. Thus, while all women are subject to the gender discourses and power relations that help to produce and sustain eating disorders, gendered abuse can accentuate contradictory and oppressive discourses so that they are deeply inscribed at an emotional level and food becomes a solution, although a similarly conflicted one. Importantly, this analysis illustrates that the ways abuse plays into an eating disorder are also highly diverse and that universal explanations are therefore limited because they cannot incorporate this. In contrast, attending to the particular socio-historical contexts framing individual women's experiences of abuse and eating disorders, including attention to gender as well as race and class, can produce a much more nuanced understanding of emotional distress that, at the same time, situates it within the wider social power relations as they manifest in particular lives.

This chapter has shown how the multiple social discourses and practices con-stituting abuse are framed by gender as well as by race and class, and how in turn these produce socially situated, gendered feelings of shame, guilt, anger, sadness and self-contempt that can play out in eating disorders in diverse ways. The chapter has also drawn attention to the dangers inherent in psychological trauma discourses of eating disorders, particularly the way they individualise, totalise and pathologise emotion and detach it from its specific social context. Nevertheless, acknowledgement of the role of abuse in eating disorders can help women challenge unequal power relations in their lives by enabling them to name their experiences *as* abuse and therefore as unacceptable. Some of the women whose interviews have been presented here also talked about overcoming emotional distress and their associated eating problems, and their experiences offer important insights into recovery from eating disorders in contexts of abuse. For example, where mainstream eating disorder treatments place an emphasis on weight and food, as well as individual psychotherapy to address emotional dis-tress, many of the women who had recovered placed an emphasis on the import-ance of unconditional relationships in their lives. Thus, just as relationships had been central to the development of an eating disorder for these women, so they were pivotal to overcoming it, too. Chapter 8 will consider the women's stories of recovery from eating disorders in the context of histories of abuse, particu-larly exploring how the exercise of interpersonal power in safe and supportive relationships became central to their mental health and wellbeing. Some of the women also mentioned abusive partners and how these experiences fed into feel-ings of low self-worth and mental health problems. The next chapter moves on to specifically examine mental health problems in the context of domestic violence.

References

American Psychiatric Association (APA) (2013) *Diagnostic and Statistical Manual of Mental Disorders – DSM-5*. Arlington: APA.

Arnow, B.A., Blasey, C.M., Hunkeler, E.M., Lee, J. and Hayward, C. (2011) Does gender modify the relationship between childhood maltreatment and adult depression? *Childhood Maltreatment*, pp. 1–9.

Bell, R.M. (1985) *Holy Anorexia*. Chicago: University of Chicago Press.

Bernstein, D.P. and Fink, L. (1998) *Childhood Trauma Questionnaire: A Retrospective Self-Report*. San Antonio: The Psychological Corporation.

Birrell, P.J. and Freyd, J.J. (2006). Betrayal trauma: relational models of harm and healing. *Journal of Trauma Practice*, 5(1), pp. 49–63.

Bordo, S. (1988) Anorexia nervosa: psychopathology as the crystallization of culture. In I. Diamond and L. Quinby (eds), *Feminism and Foucault: Reflections on Resistance*. Boston: Northeastern University Press, pp. 46–59.

Bordo, S. (1990) Reading the slender body. In M. Jacobus, E.F. Keller and S. Shuttleworth (eds), *Body/Politics: Women and the Discourses of Science*. New York: Routledge, pp. 83–112.

Bordo, S. (2009) Not just 'a white girl's thing': the changing face of food and body image problems. In H. Malson and M. Burns (eds), *Critical Feminist Approaches to Eating Dis/Orders*. Hove: Routledge, pp. 46–59.

Briere, J. and Runtz, M. (1993) Child sexual abuse, *Journal of Interpersonal Violence*, 8(3), pp. 312–330.

Bruch, H. (1974) *Eating Disorders: Obesity, Anorexia Nervosa, and the Person Within*. London: Routledge and Kegan Paul Ltd.

Bruch, H. (1978) *The Golden Cage: The Enigma of Anorexia Nervosa*. Cambridge, MA: Harvard University Press.

Budden, A. (2009) The role of shame in posttraumatic stress disorder: a proposal for a socio-emotional model for DSM-V, *Social Science & Medicine*, 69, pp. 1032–1039.

Bulbeck, C. (1998) *Social Sciences in Australia: Inequalities of Class*, second edition. Sydney: Harcourt Brace.

Burman, E., Alldred, P., Bewley, C., Goldberg, B., Heenan, C., Marks, D., Marshall, J., Taylor, K., Ullah, R. and Warner, S. (1996) *Challenging Women: Psychology's Exclusions, Feminist Possibilities*. Buckingham: Open University Press.

Crawford, J., Kippax, S., Onyx, J., Gault, U. and Benton, P. (1992) *Emotion and Gender: Constructing Meaning from Memory*. London: Sage Publications.

Crisp, A.H. (1980) *Anorexia Nervosa: Let Me Be*. London: Academic Press.

Deep, A.L., Lilenfeld, L.R., Plotnicov, K.H., Pollice, C. and Kaye, W.H. (1999) Sexual abuse in eating disorder subtypes and control women: the role of comorbid substance dependence in bulimia nervosa, *International Journal of Eating Disorders*, 25(1), pp. 1–10.

Downs, W.R. and Miller, B.A. (1998) Relationships between experiences of parental violence during childhood and women's psychiatric symptomatology, *Journal of Interpersonal Violence*, 13, pp. 438–457.

Fairburn, C.G., Marcus, M.D. and Wilson, G.T. (1993) Cognitive-behavioural therapy for binge eating and bulimia nervosa: a comprehensive treatment manual. In C.G. Fairburn and G.T. Wilson (eds), *Binge Eating: Nature, Assessment, and Treatment*. New York: The Guilford Press, pp. 361–404.

Finkelhor, D. (1994) The international epidemiology of child sexual abuse, *Child Abuse and Neglect*, 18, pp. 409–417.

Finkelhor, D. and Berliner, L. (1995) Research on the treatment of sexually abused children: a review and recommendations, *Journal of the American Academy of Child and Adolescent Psychiatry*, 34(11), pp. 1408–1423.

Fleming, J.M. (1997) Prevalence of childhood sexual abuse in a community sample of Australian women, *Medical Journal of Australia*, 166(2), pp. 65–68.

Freyd, J.J. (1997) II: violations of power, adaptive blindness and betrayal trauma theory. *Feminism and Psychology*, 7(1), pp. 22–32.

Gavey, N. (2005) *Just Sex? The Cultural Scaffolding of Rape*. Hove: Routledge.

Gavey, N. and Schmidt, J. (2011) 'Trauma of rape' discourse: a double-edged template for everyday understandings of the impact of rape? *Violence Against Women*, 17, pp. 433–456.

Goldsmith, R.E., Barlow, M.R. and Freyd, J.J. (2004) Knowing and not knowing about trauma: implications for psychotherapy, *Psychotherapy: Theory, Research, Practice, Training*, 41, pp. 448–463.

Gorton, K. (2007) Theorizing emotion and affect: feminist engagements, *Feminist Theory*, 8, pp. 333–348.

Gremillion, H. (1992) Psychiatry as social ordering: anorexia nervosa, a paradigm, *Social Science and Medicine*, 35, pp. 57–71.

Hepworth, J. (1999) *The Social Construction of Anorexia Nervosa*. London: Sage.

Herman, J.L. (1997) *Trauma and Recovery*. New York: Basic Books.

Hoglund, C.L. and Nicholas, K.B. (1995) Shame, guilt, and anger in college students exposed to abusive family environments. *Journal of Family Violence*, 10, pp. 141–157.

Hund, A.R. and Espelage, D.L. (2006) Childhood emotional abuse and disordered eating among undergraduate females: mediating influence of alexithymia and distress, *Child Abuse and Neglect*, 30, pp. 393–407.

Jacobi, C., Hayward, C., de Zwaan, M., Kraemer, H.C. and Agras, W.S. (2004) Coming to terms with risk factors for eating disorders: application of risk terminology and suggestions for a general taxonomy, *Psychological Bulletin*, 130(1), pp. 19–65.

Jaggar, A.M. (1989) Love and knowledge: emotion in feminist epistemology. In A. Garry and M. Pearsall (eds), *Women, Knowledge and Reality: Explorations in Feminist Philosophy*. London: Unwin Hyman, pp. 129–155.

Kent, A. and Waller, G. (2000) Childhood emotional abuse and eating psychopathology, *Clinical Psychology Review*, 20(7), pp. 887–903.

Le Grange, D., Lock, J., Loeb, K. and Nicholls, D. (2010) Academy for eating disorders position paper: the role of the family in eating disorders, *International Journal of Eating Disorders*, 43(1), pp. 1–5.

Lehtinen, U. (1998) How does one know what shame is? *Hypatia*, 13(1), pp. 56–78.

Levett, A. (2003) Problems of cultural imperialism in the study of child sexual abuse. In P. Reavey and S. Warner (eds), *New Feminist Stories of Child Sexual Abuse: Sexual Scripts and Dangerous Dialogues*. London: Routledge, pp. 52–76.

Loader, P. (1998) Such a shame: a consideration of shame and shaming mechanisms in families, *Child Abuse Review*, 7, pp. 44–57.

McMahon, S. (2007) Understanding community-specific rape myths: exploring student athlete culture, *Affilia: Journal of Women and Social Work*, 22(4), pp. 357–370.

McNay, L. (2004) Situated intersubjectivity. In B. Marshall and A. Witz (eds), *Engendering the Social: Feminist Encounters with Sociological Theory*. Maidenhead: Open University Press, pp. 171–186.

MacSween, M. (1993) *Anorexic Bodies*. London: Routledge.

Malson, H. (1998) *The Thin Woman: Feminism, Post-Structuralism and the Social Psychology of Anorexia Nervosa*. London: Routledge.

May-Chahal, C. (2006) Gender and child maltreatment: the evidence base, *Social Work and Society*, 4(1), pp. 53–68.

Messman-Moore, T.L. and Garrigus, A.S. (2007) The association of child abuse and eating disorder symptomatology: the importance of multiple forms of abuse and revictimization, *Journal of Aggression, Maltreatment & Trauma*, 14(3), pp. 51–72.

Nasser, M. and Malson, H. (2009) Beyond western dis/orders: thinness and self-starvation of other-ed women. In H. Malson and M. Burns (eds), *Critical Feminist Approaches to Eating Dis/Orders*. Hove: Routledge, pp. 74–86.

O'Hagan, K.P. (1993) *Emotional and Psychological Abuse of Children*. Buckingham: Open University Press.

Oppenheimer, R., Howells, K., Palmer, R.L. and Chaloner, D.A. (1985) Adverse sexual experience in childhood and clinical eating disorders: a preliminary description, *Journal of Psychiatric Research*, 19(2–3), pp. 357–361.

Palazzoli, M.S. (1974) *Self-Starvation: From the Intrapsychic to the Transpersonal Approach to Anorexia Nervosa*. London: Human Context Books.

Pelcovitz, D., Kaplan, S., Goldenberg, B., Mandel, F., Lehane, J. and Guarrera, J. (1994) Post-traumatic stress disorder in physically abused adolescents, *Journal of the American Academy of Child and Adolescent Psychiatry*, 33(3), pp. 305–312.

Potter, J. (1996) *Representing Reality: Discourse, Rhetoric and Social Construction*. London: Sage.

Probyn, E. (2005) *Blush: Faces of Shame*. Minneapolis: University of Minnesota Press.

Reay, D. (1997) Feminist theory, habitus, and social class: disrupting notions of classlessness, *Women's Studies International Forum*, 20(2), pp. 225–233.

Riessman, C.K. (2008) *Narrative Methods for the Human Sciences*. Thousand Oaks: Sage.

Root, M.P.P. and Fallon, P. (1989) Treating the victimized bulimic: the functions of binge-purge behaviour, *Journal of Interpersonal Violence*, 4(1), pp. 90–100.

Rorty, M. and Yager, J. (1996) Speculations on the role of childhood abuse in the development of eating disorders among women. In M.F. Schwartz and L. Cohn (eds), *Sexual Abuse and Eating Disorders*. New York: Brunner-Routledge, pp. 23–35.

Sayers, J. (2009) Feeding the body. In H. Malson and M. Burns (eds), *Critical Feminist Approaches to Eating Dis/Orders*. Hove: Routledge, pp. 22–34.

Scher, C.D., Ford, D.R., McQuaid, J.R. and Steen, M.B. (2004) Prevention and demographic correlates of childhood maltreatment in an adult community sample, *Child Abuse and Neglect*, 28, pp. 167–180.

Scott, S. (2001) Surviving selves: feminist and contemporary discourses of child sexual abuse, *Feminist Theory*, 2, pp. 349–361.

Sedgewick, E.K. and Frank, A. (1995) Shame in the cybernetic fold: reading Sylvan Tomkins, *Critical Inquiry*, 21(2), p. 496.

Spelman, E.V. (1989) Anger and subordination. In A. Garry and M. Pearsall (eds), *Women, Knowledge and Reality: Explorations in Feminist Philosophy*. London: Unwin Hyman, pp. 263–273.

Streigel-Moore, R.H. and Cachelin, F.M. (2001) Etiology of eating disorders in women, *The Counselling Psychologist*, 29, pp. 635–661.

Taylor, S. and Littleton, K. (2006) Biographies in talk: a narrative-discursive approach, *Qualitative Sociology Review*, 11(1), pp. 22–38.

Turner, B. (1992) *Regulating Bodies: Essays in Medical Sociology*. London: Routledge.

Walkerdine, V., Lucey, H. and Melody, J. (2001) *Growing Up Girl: Psycho-Social Explorations of Gender and Class*. London: Palgrave.

Warin, M. (2010) *Abject Relations: Everyday Worlds of Anorexia*. New Brunswick: Rutgers University Press.

Warner, S. (2009) *Understanding the Effects of Child Sexual Abuse: Feminist Revolutions in Theory, Research and Practice*. Hove: Routledge.

Weedon, C. (1987) *Feminist Practice and Poststructuralist Theory*. Oxford: Basil Blackwell.

Williams, R. (1977) *Marxism and Literature*. Oxford: Oxford University Press.

Wooley, S. (1994) Sexual abuse and eating disorders: the concealed debate. In P. Fallon, M. Katzman and S. Wooley (eds), *Feminist Perspectives on Eating Disorders*. New York: Guilford, pp. 171–211.

Wooley, S. (1996) Recognition of sexual abuse: progress and backlash. In M.F. Schwartz and L. Cohen (eds) *Sexual Abuse and Eating Disorders*. New York: Brunner-Routledge, pp. 191–209.

6 Domestic violence and emotional wellbeing

Research into the impact of domestic violence on women's mental health has increased over the last two decades. While the second wave feminist movement was instrumental in garnering attention to domestic violence more generally, as noted earlier, feminist researchers and activists were cautious about focusing on its mental health effects because of the risk of medicalisation and a shift away from justice concerns (Humphreys and Thiara, 2003). They were correct to be concerned because while there has been increased attention to mental health and domestic violence since that time, much of the research and intervention has focused on identifying the mental illnesses women suffer as a result of domestic violence as if they are detached from the experience of the violence itself. As a result, there has been little systematic attention to how gender plays out in women's understandings and experiences of themselves and their lives during and after domestic violence. The focus of this chapter is the mixed methods study into domestic violence and mental health outlined in Chapter 3.[1] Analysis of women's narratives and experiences aimed to look beyond psychiatric labels to gain insight into women's everyday lived experiences of mental health problems related to domestic violence while, at the same time, attending to how discourses about gender, domestic violence and mental illness frame women's narratives. As part of this, the chapter explores how attention might be shifted away from what is 'wrong' with women as a result of violence to what abusive men do and how this plays out psychologically and emotionally in women's lives.

Domestic violence and coercive control

Before considering the above-mentioned research, it is first useful to visit what is meant by 'domestic violence'. A widely used definition defines domestic violence as 'the patterned and repeated use of coercive and controlling behaviour to limit, direct, and shape a partner's thoughts, feelings and actions' (Almeida and Durkin, 1999: 313), involving physical, psychological/emotional, sexual, social, financial and spiritual abuse, threats and intimidation, and the use of children and pets (DeKeseredy, 2011). As noted in Chapter 2, the most salient feature of domestic violence is that it is much more likely to be perpetrated by men against women than vice versa, and involves more frequent and more injurious violence for women that has debilitating psychological consequences (Johnson *et al.*, 2014). Domestic violence has also been called 'intimate terrorism' (Johnson, 2011) or a pattern of 'coercive control' (Stark, 2007) in an effort to centre its ongoing, controlling dimensions. Stark's (2007, 2012) concept of coercive control is highly relevant to the research that myself and my colleagues have conducted into domestic violence and mental health because many of the women described experiences that are consistent with this. Stark (2012) defines coercive control as:

> an ongoing pattern of domination by which male abusive partners primarily interweave repeated physical and sexual violence with intimidation, sexual degradation, isolation and control. The primary outcome of coercive control is a condition of entrapment that can be hostage-like in the harms it inflicts on dignity, liberty, autonomy and personhood as well as to physical and psychological integrity.
>
> (Stark, 2012: 7)

Coercive control is also described as involving:

> a malevolent course of conduct that subordinates women to an alien will by violating their physical integrity (violence), denying them response and autonomy (intimidation), depriving them of social connectedness (social isolation) and appropriating or denying the resources required for personhood and citizenship.
>
> (Stark, 2007: 15)

Stark (2007) makes the case that coercive control has become more common since women have successfully secured a host of social and economic opportunities since the 1970s. There is some evidence that greater gender equality in relationships puts women at increased risk of violence by their partners (Kalmuss and Straus, 1982, cited in Walby *et al.*, 2014; O'Brien, 1975, cited in Walby, 1990). However, these connections remain unclear (Walby *et al.*, 2014). Nonetheless, Stark (2007) links controlling forms of male violence to men's efforts to retain control over women in the face of (usually overestimated) shifts in gender power relations. These changes, he argues, have led some men to find other ways of securing and enforcing their masculine privileges beyond or in addition to outright physical violence. However, in a contradictory way, while women's improved position is seen as putting them at risk of gendered violence and coercive control, their 'position in the social structure' and continued relative inequality is also understood to render them vulnerable (Stark, 2007: 16). Stark therefore argues that coercive control actively seeks to curtail women's agency and autonomy by seeking to impose a hyper-femininity that services the male partner, and that brings him social and material benefits (Stark, 2007, 2012). While it is difficult to estimate the prevalence of coercive control, Stark (2007) reports on a US study which showed that at least 60 per cent of men arrested for domestic violence in the United States had taken their partners' money as well as physically assaulted them, and that more than half had restricted their partners in other ways as well.

Domestic violence and mental health

In Chapter 2, I briefly overviewed some of the findings from psycho-medical research that links domestic violence and mental health problems in women. The large population study undertaken by myself and my colleagues asked women about the impact of domestic violence on their psychological and emotional wellbeing. Before outlining these key findings, it is useful to provide some background on the women who answered the survey and participated in the interviews. The total sample of women responding to the survey numbered 732 and included women from all around Australia, including cities, rural towns and remote areas. This research is based on a community sample, recruited through advertisements in newspapers around the country and through promotion by support services. As such, it draws on a highly diverse sample of women, particularly in terms of class. Most women were aged between 25 and 64 years of age, and most were either divorced (50.6 per cent), or re-partnered (31.4 per cent), and most of the women had children (79 per cent). A large proportion of the women were born in Australia (81.2 per cent), with 2.9 per cent women reporting Aboriginal or Torres Strait Islander backgrounds. More than half of the women (60 per cent) earned in the lower income ranges but most women had completed post-secondary education. To put the women's responses into context, the majority of violent partners were male (96.8 per cent), with women reported experiencing domestic violence from one to seven years, with an average of 3.25 years. Most women reported that they were no longer experiencing violence (82.4 per cent), and 17.3 per cent reported that they were experiencing domestic violence when they completed the survey. Half of the women reported experiencing continued violence from ex-partners after leaving, on average for 2.78 years, with one women reporting post-separation violence for 25 years. Most women reported experiencing emotional/psychological abuse (98.4 per cent) and social abuse (94.1 per cent), and 91.5 per cent of women reported physical abuse. Almost two-thirds reported sexual abuse (65.2 per cent), and a large proportion also reported financial abuse (79 per cent). Spiritual abuse was the least commonly experienced at 32.2 per cent of the women. Nonetheless, multiple types of abuse were commonly reported.

Just over half (51.5 per cent) of the women reported having received a diagnosis of a mental health problem, with nearly half (44.1 per cent) reporting depression and 41.2 per cent reporting anxiety, including PTSD and panic disorder. Only very small numbers of women reported bipolar disorder, personality or psychotic disorders. Just over a third of the women reporting a mental illness (34.4 per cent) identified multiple mental health problems, mainly anxiety and depression. Most of the women received a diagnosis of mental illness either during (42.7 per cent) or after (44.2 per cent) experiencing domestic violence, with only 13 per cent reporting receiving a diagnosis before domestic violence. Thus, most women received a diagnosis either while still in domestic violence or after leaving. A significant proportion of women answered the question asking them to rate their psychological and mental health before, during and after domestic violence (N=613). Almost three-quarters of this group (70 per cent) indicated good psychological and emotional wellbeing before domestic violence, while 90 per cent reported poor psychological and emotional wellbeing during violence and 65 per cent reported poor mental health afterwards. A further question asked women to rate their psychological wellbeing on a five-point scale (1 = very poor; 2 = poor; 3 = fair; 4 = good; 5 = very good). Before domestic violence, women's mean rating of their wellbeing was 4.00 (SD = 1.02) (i.e. 'good'); during domestic violence their mean rating was 1.45 (SD = 0.68) (i.e. 'very poor' to 'poor'); immediately after leaving the violent situation, the women's mean rating had risen slightly to 2.33 (SD = 1.52) (i.e. 'poor') and; current mean wellbeing was reported at 3.27 (SD = 1.53) (i.e. 'fair'). These differences were statistically significant (F $(1,597)=309.22$, p<0.001). These figures show that many women do not consider themselves to have bounced back in terms of emotional wellbeing even though they had left the violent relationship. Most of the women (84 per cent) reported they had had contact with a professional about their psychological and emotional wellbeing. In spite of many women reporting poorer mental health as a result of domestic violence, many nonetheless reported feeling hopeful about their future (44.8 per cent) or not discouraged about their future (17.2 per cent) while, concerningly, 17.6 per cent reported that they feel discouraged about the future and a further 13.3 per cent reported they do not expect things to work out and that the future is hopeless and will get worse.

While this chapter is focused on domestic violence and mental health, the research study conducted with my colleagues also demonstrated the significant impact of violence on other dimensions of women's lives, specifically employment and housing, and these are not unrelated to mental health. Before experiencing intimate partner violence (IPV), 50.2 per cent of women were in full-time employment, 14.6 per cent part-time employment and 9.1 per cent casual employment. At the time of completing the survey, under a third were in full-time employment (29.6 per cent), 18.8 per cent were in part-time employment and 16.3 per cent were unemployed or not seeking work (16.3 per cent). Before experiencing domestic violence, 8.2 per cent reported full-time home duties. At the time of completing the survey, the proportion of women reporting home duties (16.7 per cent) had doubled. Thus, the numbers of women in full-time employment dropped significantly, with implications for income levels. Most women were currently in the lower income ranges, with 40 per cent earning under $30,000 pa, 13.7 per cent earning $30,000–$39,000 pa, and 10 per cent earning $40,000–$49,000 pa. Most women also reported that they lived in a jointly owned house (42.2 per cent) or in a private rental property (36.3 per cent) before leaving domestic violence, but at the time of completing the survey, the majority of women reported living in a private rental property (40.3 per cent) or were sole owners of a house (20.7 per cent). Thus, the rate of home ownership had fallen dramatically. Domestic violence therefore had a dramatic impact on the material conditions of women's lives, and some women perceived this as worsening their struggles with mental health.

In the remainder of this chapter, I present an analysis of women's narratives about the impact of domestic violence on their psychological and emotional wellbeing drawn from the large mixed methods study mentioned earlier. Using the concept of situated intersubjectivity (McNay, 2004), I explore the impact of violence on women's sense of self and identity by considering how violence and mental illness are discursively constructed in language and how these play out in women's lived experiences of mental health problems, particularly their emotional dimensions. Thus, I aim to take a step beyond simple linear conceptualisations of a causal relationship between domestic violence and mental illness to a more critical appraisal of how symbolic and material processes of engendering frame women's narratives and experiences. The following analysis of qualitative data from the survey and interviews sits under two main overarching themes:

1   regimes of gendered control; and
2   gendered violence and gender identities.

The first theme maps out the types of abuse experienced by the women as the backdrop to their specific experiences of emotional distress with the aim of seeking to closely connect women's experiences of violence with their experiences of mental health problems. The second theme focuses on teasing out the different dimensions of the impact of domestic violence on women's mental health, demonstrating how closely these mirror the intent of gendered violence and coercive control.

Gender, self and identity in violence-related mental health problems

The analysis presented here specifically draws on the qualitative text-based answers women offered in response to the survey question, *What impact has domestic violence had on your psychological and emotional wellbeing?*, to which 557 women responded, and the qualitative life history interviews with 17 women about their experiences of domestic violence and mental health.

Setting the context: life under regimes of gendered control

Before exploring the women's descriptions of the impact of domestic violence on their mental health, I want to paint a picture of the nature of the gendered violence they experienced. While physical violence and the threat of it was an important strategy for partners in maintaining power and control, at an everyday level the women particularly talked about high levels of emotional, sexual, financial and social abuse. These types of abuse are central to coercive control (Stark, 2007) and, as noted above, many of the women described these alongside physical violence, with most of the women experiencing multiple types. Here, I present an analysis of the women's narratives of violence and abuse, and I show how these reflect Stark's (2007) model of coercive control in many respects, although they also include additional types of abusive control not identified by Stark. All of the women whose narratives are presented here went on to describe mental health problems as a result of gendered violence and coercive control. The women's narratives provide a sense not only of the nature of the physical violence they experienced but how it under-girded other types of control and abuse.

In emphasising the role of emotional, sexual, financial and social abuse in coercive control, I do not mean to play down the extent of the physical violence described by many of the women. Women's descriptions included being punched, hit, choked, pushed and kicked, with some women reporting assaults serious enough to require hospitalisation or medical attention, while many mentioned threats of violence. Many women described quite intense feelings of fear in relation to the violence itself but also the threat of it, including in some cases fear of death. Felicia said 'he would sit there and threaten to kill me or run his finger across his throat', while Vivien described a frightening situation where she realised her partner had decided to kill her because he had discovered her plan to leave:

> I was watching to see what he was up to, and there was a knife on the bench ... and I saw him pick that up and hide it, like down the side of his body, and then he got to kind walk right behind me, and I could see by his face that he decided in that second to kill me, and he actually was sort of right behind [me] ... so I knew that I was sort of seconds away from being killed again ... and [because I then said something that indicated I wasn't leaving] you could see him doubt then that I was going to leave and again and again that happened and you could see this kind of rage and this determination that he was going to kill me, and the only thing that stopped him was the doubt that I was going to leave.
>
> (Vivien)

In Vivien's account, her partner's decision to murder her is predicated on his perception that she was about to leave. The threat of physical violence was therefore experienced by Vivien as controlling and dictating her decisions and movements. This controlling dimension of the threat of violence was most succinctly captured by Sheila in her survey response when she explained in a sardonic tone that there was only 'occasional violence [because] I was very obedient and didn't need much beyond a threat to refocus me'. As observed by Stark (2007), actual physical violence is often in the background to other forms of gendered control and abuse.

One of the most common experiences the women described was their partners' use of verbal put-downs and name-calling. Veronica talked about experiencing 'lots and lots of control, running me down all the time', while Lizzie said:

He would deride me all the time.... He would build me up – call me names, terrible. I can tell you what they were if you want? A 'fucking retarded slut', 'expensive pet to keep' he would tell people, 'she's a very expensive pet to keep'. Whereas I was earning as much if not more than him.

(Lizzie)

Verbal denigration also involved scapegoating women, with a number of the women describing being routinely blamed by partners, including for his own abusive behaviour. As part of verbal denigration, many women also specifically described being called 'mentally unstable' by their partners, commonly after the men's violence and control had caused them psychological distress, which was then used by the men to further justify their abuse. This has been widely identified in other studies, too (for example, Laing and Toivonen, 2010). Some women described their partners explicitly seeking to paint them as mad and unreliable to the rest of the world, including their families, friends, the courts, and health and welfare agencies. The verbal denigration described here therefore had a distinctly gendered flavour, drawing on a range of femininity discourses. Hence, Lizzie was accused of (female) irrationality/stupidity, sexual promiscuity and dependency as 'an expensive pet'; scapegoating sought to shift responsibility for abuse onto women themselves and away from abusers; and accusations of mental instability drew on the long-standing historical discourses that associate femininity with madness (Showalter, 1987), thereby discrediting the women's opinions and distress.

A further common tactic of gendered control described by the women involved the manipulation and use of children by violent partners. This practice has received increasing attention from researchers and practitioners in recent years but was not specifically identified by Stark (2007) in his model of coercive control. Some women described their partners blaming them for the children's behaviour, a further form of scapegoating that is also highly gendered because it is predicated on discourses that position mothers as primarily responsible for children. Other women talked about their partners' use of tactics of maternal alienation (Morris, 1999). Sascha described the following situation:

From the time I left there was this ongoing campaign of maternal alienation to tell the kids how stupid I was and it just went on and on and on and on. And it definitely affected my relationship with the kids and it upset them a lot.

(Sascha)

She went on to say, 'he started this unbelievable amount of revenge behaviour. He'd kidnap my children for a week and I wouldn't know where they were'. Evelyn described being unable to leave because of her partner's dictum that she could not take her son with her: 'I tried to leave him a couple of times in the past but always got too scared to go and he always said that I couldn't take [my son] with me.' May talked about her partner making death threats in relation to the children:

He said that I would do as I was told or else he would kill the kids. And so I was very protective of the kids and [my son] never understood why I would drop him off to school while everyone else walks.

(May)

Other women described child custody battles based on the men's desire for revenge for leaving rather than a genuine desire to be with and care for their children. Previous research has also reported men's use of children as a revenge tactic, sometimes ending with the men murdering the children (Johnson, 2005). Attacking women through their children is specifically gendered because it strikes at a key domain of femininity and feminine agency for many women in its focus on mothering. In recent research conducted by myself and my colleagues, we show how women go to great lengths to protect their children from violent partners. This included scheduling activities in ways that will reduce outbursts of violence, taking the blame and complying with partners' unreasonable demands to keep the peace and protect children, and developing safety plans with children for when violence erupts (Moulding *et al.*, 2015; Buchanan *et al.*, 2014).

Many women also described the widely noted control tactic of social isolation from family and friends (for example, Stark, 2007). Mariana said 'he was trying to isolate me ... he didn't want me to Skype my family.... He started saying, "oh you cannot Skype your family"'. May said:

The first thing he did was isolate me. So he got me away from the family and every time I would make friends in a new town we would move.... I would make friends, we would move. I'd make friends, we'd move. I'd make friends, we'd move.

(May)

Freya also said:

It took a long time to remember how to socialise, because he didn't let me have friends, he would get jealous and, very jealous. One occasion where I went to see a movie with some friends from Uni, just two girls, later when I mentioned I'd seen the movie he was like 'Oh yeah, who did you go with again?' Jealous. And it just – they beat you down in a way in which you think you can't socialise with people, and they tell you you're doing everything wrong, and it takes a long while to learn how to talk to people again.

(Freya)

As is pointed out by Stark (2007), social isolation increases the male partner's control over their female partners. Women also described control tactics focused on the management of their appearance, weight and sexuality. The following extract from Felicia further captures this:

I didn't even realise just how bad things were actually getting because it was so gradual. Like in the beginning it was 'Oh you can't wear that because it makes you a slut. Why do you have make up on? Who are you trying to impress?' And things were just so gradual that by the end I wasn't allowed to see any friends, wasn't allowed to go anywhere, do anything without him accusing me of cheating … you don't even realise it's happening.

(Felicia)

Felicia described her partner controlling what she wore based on his fear that she was trying to attract other men. One woman even described her partner preventing her from going to the gym for fear she might attract men through having a fit body! In the next account, Veronica described her partner's accusations of infidelity and constant monitoring of her whereabouts through phone calls:

He kept phoning me at first and saying that I've got another boyfriend, that I'm pregnant to someone else, all these…. Everything was my fault. [He] accused me of having affairs with my boss or anyone else who called, that was kind of his angle but he did not worry about me having a job because I paid all the bills.

(Veronica)

Harassment of the women through calls and texting to check up on their whereabouts was extremely common and is also identified in Stark's research (2007). Also in common with Stark's (2007) studies, some women described their partners checking their computers and mobile phones to see who they had been in contact with, and a couple of women even described their partners or ex-partners secretly installing listening devices and surveillance cameras in their houses. Many women also mentioned being stalked by the partners both while they were in the relationship but particularly after they had left. Much of this behaviour was presented by the women as particularly marked and driven by obsessive concern and jealousy about imagined sexual relations with other men. In fact, this was a central and distinctive feature of the abuse many of the women described.

While having a job could invite high levels of monitoring, surveillance and control from violent partners, it could also bring financial exploitation and abuse. Veronica said that her partner was happy for her to work because 'he enjoyed the fruits of my labour'. Many women talked about their partners taking the money they earned and tightly controlling their spending. In contrast, other women described being banned from working because they would be generally outside their partners' scrutiny during work hours and potentially in the company of other men. Control tactics also focused on women's domestic responsibilities, an observation emphasised by Stark (2007) who argues that this further underscores the gendered nature of coercive control as an attack on feminine agency. Freya explained:

He started to get angry at me for the house being messy, and I said well hold on … you constantly want my attention when you're home. So if I get up to do the dishes you say 'Leave it' and yeah, it was just, he would constantly try to interrupt me cleaning the house, and then have a reason to yell at me … it'd be snide remarks, sort of, more like 'What have you been doing all day?' 'You've been home all day, what have you been doing, why isn't the house clean if you've been nothing all day?'

(Freya)

Some women in the interviews not uncommonly described retaining all or most of the responsibility for domestic chores and child-care, even when they were in paid work and their partners were not. These women were usually in socially disadvantaged families where the men were involved with drugs, demonstrating the intersection of class with gender in women's explanations and experiences of gendered violence. While some of the men tolerated their partners working because of the economic benefits it brought them, many were not so supportive of the women's efforts to study. Sascha said:

He threw all my books out the window and every time I had an assignment due … every time there was an assignment due he would have some, there would be some gigantic argument, the violence was huge when … I was at university the violence was enormous.

Q: OK, so this was perceived as a great threat?
A: It definitely was, yeah.

(Sascha)

Freya not dissimilarly said:

Once we moved in there was, quite early on, signs that things weren't quite right … like, he seemed very jealous of the fact that I was studying at the time … he was very jealous that I'd had the opportunity to go to Uni … in the beginning it was just, I would have my notes out on the coffee table in the lounge room just, because I'd been at Uni just trying to consolidate all my notes and get everything together. He'd come home from work, I'd offer to make him a coffee or a tea or dinner or whatever, and in the meantime, while I'm in the kitchen trying to get something for him, he'd throw my notes on the floor and say 'Why are you making such a fucking mess?'

(Freya)

Freya went on to explain that the reason she failed to complete her university degree was because 'he wouldn't let me leave the house until it was clean, but every time he got home he would mess it up and it just became a vicious cycle'. Thus, Freya described her partner virtually imprisoning her through housework so that the requirement to undertake never-ending domestic chores effectively stopped her from gaining a degree and a career in law. This speaks to another important element of the coercive control described by the women that is similarly emphasised by Stark (2007): the control tactics (and violence) escalated when the women attempted to better themselves, became more independent or when the men realised they were planning to leave. Earlier, Vivien described her realisation that her partner meant to kill her on discovering her plan to leave, while Lizzie mentioned her partner calling her 'an expensive pet' when she earned more than him. Veronica said:

> He quit jobs and was unemployed for chunks of time do you know what I mean? He enjoyed the fruits of my labour. So that was not an issue for him although I'm sure the power imbalance that it caused ... contributed to his actions or his attitudes so while on one hand he was quite happy for me to work and to spend my money, let's put it frankly but he was certainly jealous. He didn't like me to talk about my work at all.
>
> (Veronica)

Thus, Veronica's experience led her to conclude that the power imbalance brought on by her working contributed to jealousy on her partner's part and increased efforts to control her. Gertrude specifically explained how her partner's controlling behaviour increased when she began to become more independent once the children had grown:

> The domestic violence didn't really start till about the last three or four years and it sort of coincided with me becoming more independent.... I was elected to a [local] council and he really resented that because I loved it. Part of it was very stressful later on but I found it really stimulating. He was OK with me going to the young wives' clubs and mothers and babies type functions when the kids were little. That was no threat to him. But with this other one I was going to meetings with fellow members, mainly men, at night and he started thinking I was having it off with them, very jealous and it just escalated from there.
>
> (Gertrude)

Gertrude believed that her husband's jealousy about her being in the company of other men and his ungrounded fears of her infidelity was the main driving force behind the increase in his controlling behaviour. Evelyn described how her partner became physically and sexually violent when he realised she was planning to leave:

> As soon as he got wind that I was making the noises to leave ... that's when he first started getting physically violent. He was a bit rough in bed, is how it started. Just wanting to bring bondage into the relationship and just getting, just rough that way.
>
> (Evelyn)

The use of rape and other types of sexual violence was a reasonably common experience reported by the women: almost two-thirds of the women in the survey sample (65 per cent) indicated sexual violence. Gertrude linked a rape perpetrated by her partner to his perception that she was becoming too independent, explaining how 'it was just the slaps and the push and the emotional abuse … [but the rape] happened in the last year when he felt as if he was losing complete control of me'. Not dissimilarly, May said:

> That was the funny thing. I thought I had found Mr Perfect. And this one night we were out dancing and someone asked me to dance and I was dancing with him and I noticed a change in mood, but when I got home he started both raping me and slapping me across the face.
>
> Q: Because you were dancing with someone else?
> A: Because I was dancing with someone else and he said that I hadn't asked permission, and I remember lying there and thinking 'is this happening?' I was in shock.

(May)

The tactics described by the women therefore reflect Stark's (2007) model in important ways. However, the women also drew attention to additional forms of gendered abuse such as scapegoating and control through the abuse and manipulation of children. Taken together, the controlling tactics described by the women were largely concerned with the enforcement of a compliant, servile femininity (Stark, 2007). Moreover, where women were allowed to participate in the workforce in line with more contemporary gender expectations, they often presented this as for the men's own financial gain that nonetheless seemed to challenge their masculine identities. While many of these controlling tactics revolved around the imposition of a traditional femininity, many also often involved undermining women in what is nonetheless a key field of feminine agency and identity – the domestic realm – adding further complexity to the negative impact on women.

While Stark (2007) elaborates the controlling nature of domestic violence, he gives only passing attention to the mental health consequences of this for women. As outlined earlier, other research shows that domestic violence is strongly associated with negative mental health outcomes for women, such as PTSD, anxiety and depression, but Stark insists that only a small proportion of women actually evidence these problems. He suggests that this is because most assaults are too minor to induce trauma and he then sets out to demonstrate the important ways that women exercise agency and ingenuity in the face of coercive control. Stark's treatment of the question of the impact of domestic violence and coercive control on mental health is also at times contradictory because, after arguing that few women actually manifest conditions such as PTSD, he also states that many do experience mental health problems. Stark has a specific interest in women who go on to kill their partners, and in seeking to show that they are not 'the hapless victim who have eventually cracked', as they are often depicted in medical defence cases, the more general question of the effects of violence and control on mental health is brushed over. More specifically, Stark seems to remain within a gendered and medicalised understanding of mental health and illness that offers only two positions: that abused women are mentally ill victims and therefore irrational, or that abused women are not mentally ill and therefore agentic, and it is the second of these that he takes up. This is based on a limited, binary theorisation of gender and mental illness. It is also based on a rather narrow, structuralist understanding of gender and violence. Anderson (2009) argues that Stark mainly aims to demonstrate how structural gender inequality provides men with the ability to deploy coercive control and that he therefore gives little attention to gender identity and the interactional dimensions of gender in the everyday. There is a large body of feminist theorisation relevant to this that has potential for offering a deeper, more nuanced understanding of the impact of domestic violence on mental health, and I engage with this later to help make sense of women's experiences of violence-related mental health problems. First, though, I present the following analysis of women's narratives of gendered violence and mental health problems, seeking to locate their explanations and experiences in the specific context of the gendered violence and coercive control described above.

Gendered violence, gender identities and mental health

The interviews and the open-ended survey question about the impact of domestic violence on women's psychological and emotional wellbeing provided important insights into women's understandings and lived experiences of poor mental health during and after violence. In common with the quantitative data from this study and the wider research literature in this area, most women reported the development of mental health problems, with PTSD, anxiety and depression the most often mentioned. Many women also mentioned experiencing panic, insomnia, difficulty concentrating, flashbacks, nightmares, feeling numb, substance abuse, suicidal feelings and fear of raised voices, particularly male voices, alongside feelings of low self-worth, low self-esteem, low self-confidence, fear, grief, exhaustion and sadness. Most importantly, and as shown in other studies (for example, Humphreys and Thiara, 2003), the women drew a direct causal relationship between their experiences of domestic violence and their subsequent struggles with mental health. In addition to this, some women were also able to offer rich insights into the impact of violence and coercive control on their sense of themselves, their identities, their social relations with others and their sense of place in the world. In these instances, they tended not to use medical or psychological language, and such accounts were particularly offered in response to the open-ended survey question about emotional wellbeing. This perhaps reflects the anonymous nature of the online survey method and the protection it offers from feelings of judgement or embarrassment that might be felt in the presence of an interviewer. Research participants are often emotionally self-protective in a face-to-face situation, particularly in the avoidance of shame (Probyn, 2005). This is not to say that the interviews did not yield rich insights into emotional experience too, though: the women were able to tease out in more detail how the different types of abuse impacted on their emotional wellbeing in this forum, as well as explain their resistance to depowering subjectivities.

Thematic analysis of the survey and interview data identified three main themes that constructed the different dimensions of the impact of gendered violence on women's emotional wellbeing. First, some women talked about difficulties in recognising themselves as 'victims of violence' through the theme, 'this is not me'; second, gendered violence and abuse were presented by many women as specifically leading to a lost or changed sense of self and identity; third, some women talk about becoming aware of 'an unsafe world' and a shifting sense of their place within it. The analysis will demonstrate how the women's mental health experiences mirrored in many respects the gendered control tactics used by their partners, and will explore in some detail how dominant discourses about gender and mental illness frame and further complicate this picture. I must point out here, though, that some women also talked about the positive aspects of domestic violence and coercive control in terms of making them stronger, more self-directed and assertive, more self-protective and unwilling to wear blame for others' behaviour, while others talked about regaining their sense of self or discovering new identities after leaving the violent relationship. These accounts will be considered in the following chapter: here, I am primarily concerned with theorising the emotional distress caused by gendered violence beyond the narrow confines of medical and psychological discourses, as well as with elaborating the gender and psychological discourses women drew on to explain their experiences. Quite a few women also identified physical health problems as a result of gendered violence, such as chronic pain. While such conditions were often presented as tied up with their mental health (Nicolaidis *et al.*, 2008), I have specifically focused only on the latter.

'This is not me': disrupted identities and gendered violence

In this section, I consider women's narratives of identity – the ways they described their sense of themselves – in the context of violence and coercive control. Many women specifically described the impact of domestic violence on their perceptions of, and feelings about, themselves and some also reflected on how this compared with their self-identities before domestic violence. It is important to remember that almost three-quarters (70 per cent) of the sample of 613 women who answered this question indicated good psychological and emotional wellbeing before domestic violence, with only 13 per cent reporting a diagnosis of mental illness prior to the violent relationship. The narratives of those women who made comments about their identities before and after violence crudely fell into two main groups. In the first, and smaller, group some women described struggling with mental health problems prior to domestic violence, mentioning histories of child abuse, child sexual abuse or growing up in domestic violence. These women also described low self-confidence and feelings of worthlessness prior to the violent relationship, which then seemed to confirm their sense of worthlessness and of deserving bad treatment. Domestic violence and coercive control therefore seemed to reinforce for some women a pre-existing sense of worthlessness and negative identity wrought by previous gendered violence and abuse. Other research studies into re-victimisation confirm that histories of abuse prior to domestic violence can complicate mental health problems for some women (Classen *et al.*, 2001; Humphreys and Thiara, 2003). The second, and larger, group of women described themselves as quite different before and after violence, with some explicitly portraying themselves as confident, independent and sure of themselves and only struggling with mental health problems once violence began. These women tended not to identify prior histories of gendered abuse, and portrayed the realisation that they were victims of domestic violence as a grave shock that was highly disruptive to their sense of themselves. Many of the women who described themselves as changed because of domestic violence therefore drew a sharp distinction between who they felt they were before the violent relationship and who they felt they became after it:

> It reduced my self-confidence, left me fearful, sad, under-mined my belief in my ability to take care of myself. I was very self-assured and super-confident, ambitious, popular and professionally and personally successful.
>
> (Margot)

> It has changed me as a person. I am no longer the happy bubbly full of confidence person I once was.
>
> (Sally)

> I don't have the confidence I used to have. I was previously a very bubbly and positive person, highly motivated and a high achiever. Now I feel like the future is very grim for me.
>
> (Debbie)

Many of the women who described changed identities also talked about the gradual onset of abuse so that by the time they realised there was a problem, they were already trapped in the violent relationship. For example, Marilyn said 'I am a strong and intelligent woman and I can't believe I met someone like him. They are master manipulators'. Felicia expected that she would be able to 'spot it … and get out' but this did not reflect her experience of the slow burn of domestic violence and coercive control:

> Like all these common things people used to think, that people still think that I don't. Like it happened that gradual I didn't even realise it was happening. Whereas I thought, always grow up thinking if I'm ever in a

relationship like that I can easily spot it and it's easy to get out, but by the time it gets to the point where you realise it, it's too late, it's too hard to get out without help. But you're even too scared to ask for help at that stage.

(Felicia)

Other research shows that gendered violence and coercive control usually begins in an insidious manner with psychological violence and controlling behaviour that is difficult to initially identify (for example, Scheffer Lindgren and Renck, 2008). Along these lines, some women mentioned not realising that what they were experiencing could be seen as domestic violence. Amelia said 'I mean right now we see it as everything was just abusive you know, but at that time no I wouldn't have even occurred to me the word abuse or violence or anything like that'. Winona pointed out that only once the abuse was named and identified by others did it became real to her:

She [the psychologist] said I've been terribly abused for 23 years, and so that was a shock, so you don't realise that, because what I was going through I didn't realise was abuse until now, when it's all in the public eye that you realise.

(Winona)

This draws attention to the importance of naming violence and abuse. Winona's difficulty in recognising her experiences as abuse also arose in part because she was one of the few women who did not experience direct physical assault, and this was also the case for Mariana:

Because at the beginning I didn't see myself ... no, I'm not beaten or a person who's at risk, so it was a long process to say, 'oh my God, this is domestic violence'.

Q: OK, so you came to name it as that. And what difference did it make for you when you named it like that?
A: It was very shocking. Because I never ... it, so I wrote a lot about that, I interview a lot of women ... domestic violence, and to see myself in that situation it was like, you know, how stupid can you be – like, God, I mean you knew that ... and I studied that, and I wrote so much about that, and then it was, you know, like eyes opening – God.... I saw, OK yes, it's not physical but it's verbally and psychological abuse and its bullying, and I felt afraid of him ... because when he gets angry he's totally out of control.

(Mariana)

Mariana therefore expressed a level of incredulity that she did not realise she was in an abusive relationship even after she had researched and written about domestic violence as a journalist. Gertrude was not dissimilarly surprised by the fact that she had been on a panel about domestic violence as part of her council work but had not 'recognised myself at all'.

> But see on looking back the violence had virtually started before then but I just thought it was one off, a slap and a punch and then I got the carnations and the remorse and coincidentally I was on a panel as part of my duties as an elected member dealing with domestic violence but I didn't recognise myself at all.
>
> (Gertrude)

Vivien dismissed her intuition about the 'red flags' she was picking up about her partner, almost berating herself that she was 'being awful' because he 'hadn't done anything':

> I suppose the red flags sort of started to appear, and I never did get rid of that fear that something was wrong, and I'd say to myself you know, you're being awful, he hasn't done anything, but then I'd say well, you're picking something up, so there must be something.
>
> (Vivien)

Vivien's intuition later became a life-saver when she was in serious danger. As noted earlier, May talked about her complete shock when her partner raped her for dancing with other men, mistakenly thinking she had found 'Mr Perfect', while other women mentioned their partners completely changing after the early phase of the relationship. For example, Scarlett said, 'My ex-husband was so nice to me in the first two years we were together and then we got married so it all changed ... then I felt as if I kept getting hit by a truck every week'.

The fact that many of the women did not expect domestic violence and coercive control, nor recognised themselves as victims of it once it began, does not signify any special ignorance on their part. Many contemporary women implicitly assume they are equal to men and that domestic responsibilities will be mutual (Lamanna, 1999; Sharpe, 2001), although prospective partners may not necessarily share these expectations (Sharpe, 2001). Of course, this does not necessarily mean that women see themselves as the *same* as men, though, because discourses of natural gender differences are also common (Chung, 2005). However, as Chung (2005) points out, wider discourses about gender equality can work to obscure gender power relations and related gendered violence, making it difficult to recognise them as such. Violent and controlling men are also commonly very careful to present quite a different front to the woman in the early days of the relationship (Stark, 2007), as indicated by May and Scarlett above. Other studies have identified women's sense of shock when their male partners first become violent, with the men's oscillation between violence and seeking forgiveness also confusing the situation (for example, Scheffer Lindgren and Renck, 2008). In domestic violence, the abuse has also been perpetrated by the very person who is supposed to be loving and supportive, adding to both shock and shame but also to feelings of betrayal and abandonment (Freyd, 1997; Scheffer Lindgren and Renck, 2008). Moreover, jealousy and possessiveness can be misinterpreted as signs of love (Stark, 2007) within hegemonic heterosexual scripts. However, as demonstrated earlier, many of the women in this study had particularly experienced coercive control, with a small number not experiencing actual physical violence, although the threat of it was usually present. Stark (2007) argues that coercive control is 'invisible in plain sight' in the sense that it is not officially recognised despite the fact that women have been describing it for decades (Stark, 2007: 14). As demonstrated above, then, some of the women were not aware of gendered forms of coercive control until they experienced it themselves, making it difficult to name their treatment as abusive.

Because many women in this study described identities as capable women in control of their lives prior to violent or controlling relationships, it is likely that violence and control were experienced as particularly shocking and highly disruptive to their sense of themselves. The study by Scheffer Lindgren and Renck (2008) of PTSD after domestic violence not dissimilarly showed that many of the women regarded themselves as strong before domestic violence and felt severely ashamed of being manipulated and violated by controlling violent men, as well as guilty for placing themselves in such a situation. As Marilyn said above, 'I am a strong and intelligent woman, and I can't believe I met someone like him'. Women who were confident prior to violence may therefore experience themselves in particularly contradictory and confusing ways, while women who have pre-existing histories of abuse and mental health problems may have quite different reactions and perhaps deeper, more continuous feelings of worthlessness and low self-esteem.

'I am not the same person': lost sense of self and agency

Of those women who described themselves as changed by domestic violence, many said that they had lost the sense of themselves *as* selves with continuous identities, agency and autonomy. Thus, many women talked about no longer feeling like themselves, feeling empty inside or having lost their sense of self. Just over 10 per cent (n=61, 11 per cent) of the women who responded to the open-ended survey question about the impact of violence on their psychological and emotional wellbeing offered up this unprompted understanding of their experiences, and most of them described the development of specific mental health problems as a result of violence. Almost all of these women had indicated experiences of abuse that were consistent with coercive control. The phenomenon of lost sense of self and changed identity in response to violence and abuse was succinctly captured in the following comments from women's survey responses. These are selected responses from a much larger body of similar, unprompted statements referring to experiences of lost, shattered or empty selves: 'I am not the same person, the trauma of the relationship has left me a different person. It has absolutely shattered me'; 'It destroyed me mentally, physically and emotionally. I became an empty shell, completely dead inside';

'I don't even recognise myself sometimes.'; 'I feel like I will never be the same person'; 'My confidence, trust and self-esteem is gone. I am not the same person I was.' Thus, like the women who earlier described themselves as confident prior to violence, many drew a sharp distinction between who they felt they were before violence and control and who they felt they became during and after it. Elise elaborated this felt lost sense of self further:

> I feel the trauma of the relationship has left me a different person and even though it's been years since I left the abusive relationship, I feel that it has changed me and this in turn has affected my life. My confidence and self-esteem have been shattered, my social life has been dissolved, my financial situation has decreased and I feel a panic that I have fallen off the merry-go-round and can't get back on. I am also anxious in a relationship fearing that I will be hurt again.
>
> (Elise)

Elise referred here to lost self-confidence and self-esteem, as did other women earlier. Almost one-third (n = 179, 31 per cent) of the survey sample of women specifically mentioned lost self-confidence, self-esteem and self-worth as the main effects of violence and control. Self-esteem is central to an individual's sense of being able to act in the world (Lister, 2007) and is therefore pivotal to a felt capacity for agency. The following account also emphasises lost identity and self-confidence, but specifically ties this to lost freedom and autonomy:

> I lost my identity as an individual. My every movement and action was dictated by the fear of a negative reaction from former partner. I adopted the 'peace at any price' mentality. I lost my self-confidence, [developed] high levels of anxiety and depression, which he threatened to leave me over if it would be an ongoing issue.
>
> (Kiara)

Many other women referred to similar experiences of 'walking on eggshells' around their partners. While interpreting and making decisions in response to a partner's feelings and reactions requires high levels of intelligence and agency, the above account directly links this to loss of confidence, identity, anxiety and depression. Thus, needing to constantly prioritise the preferences and feelings of another because of the threat of violence and control is portrayed and experienced as dehumanising, humiliating and undermining of self-identity and confidence. This is not to suggest that monitoring and responding to the needs of others is necessarily dehumanising in and of itself: rather, it points to how tending to others' needs is denigrating when it is forced rather than chosen. Eleanor specifically talked about no longer knowing or feeling herself as a result of domestic violence, and therefore not knowing how to *be* herself in the world:

It has crushed me inside … every day is a struggle to get up and face the world. Then to try and look normal to my kids so they don't feed off my feelings. Every day is a challenge to just get kids ready and then go to work and then come home do household things help with homework and prepare for next day. I was once a vibrant, well-liked, sporty and social young woman. I lost 20 years of my life and now I don't know how to be me!

(Eleanor)

Eleanor points to having to hide her feelings from the world and her children behind the mask of 'the functioning mother' to conceal her violence-related struggles with day-to-day living, saying that this has led her to no longer know how to be herself, the woman she was before violence. The following account specifically draws attention to the role of self-doubt in lost sense of self and agency related to abuse:

I used to be strong-willed and positive, sure of myself and my choices. During the domestic violence I could make no choices. Now I doubt the clothes I buy and wear, the way I wear my hair and the things I say to other people. I was always told that I said the wrong thing and that I shouldn't have said whatever it was I said.

(Haley)

In this extract, self-doubt and the feeling of being 'wrong' – an accusation Haley said was levelled at her as part of verbal abuse – is contrasted with having felt strong-willed and sure of herself and her choices in the past. Feeling able to make choices is the very hallmark of human agency (Davies, 1991) and knowing what one thinks, believes and feels underpins this. As shown earlier, having to defer to the desires of another can result in women no longer knowing what they think or feel. The following comment from Tanya spelt out very clearly the effect of violence and control on knowing, believing and feeling when she said, 'I was no longer able to believe anything to be true, every belief, thought, feeling was totally questionable'. Not dissimilarly, Paige said, 'Inside I always have self-doubt and a very critical inner voice. I continually doubt myself'. Some of these accounts describe an unsettling subjectivity and reality where nothing is any longer true because all beliefs, feelings and self-identity have been brought into question. Such a state brings to mind Anthony Giddens' concept of 'ontological security', defined as:

confidence or trust that the natural or social worlds are as they appear to be, including the basic existential parameters of the self and social identity having trust that the world is as it appears to be, including self and social identity.

(Giddens, 1997, cited in Davidson, 2000: 38)

Thus, the women's accounts invoke the idea of no longer having a secure ontological base from which to operate because violence and coercive control have torn down their sense of themselves, their truths and beliefs, their desires, and their assumptions about the world.

As so powerfully and succinctly put by Amaya, 'abuse isn't just them slamming a fist in your face, it's all this stuff in your head'. In addition to losing touch with preferences and desires through deference to another, many women like Haley earlier spoke of losing their sense of self through the development of a critical inner voice that replayed their partners' abusive words in their heads, even well after they had escaped him. In the following account, Kylie talked about replaying the verbal abuse over and over in her mind and the effect this had:

> I get caught in my brain and replay and hear all the things I was called and accused of, all the threats and how I was to be murdered. I just seem to have lost my mojo over the past 13 years of hell and as much as I try I cannot regain it. I feel alone and sometimes think the shit [he] said must be true and that's why it happened. Domestic violence has made my brain weak, exposed to things I would never imagine. I believe I will never mentally be the same.
>
> (Kylie)

This account brings to mind the tactic of brain-washing in war, whereby the victim comes to believe what they are repeatedly told and loses sight of their own beliefs. Herman (1997) has illustrated how male perpetrators of child sexual abuse silence victims through this tactic, and it is also part of the coercive control of adult women in domestic violence, too (Stark, 2007). This account also reflects the observation that women more generally embody both the surveyed and the surveyor, the actor and the spectator (Showalter, 1987), with an inner (usually male) critical voice monitoring a woman's appearance and all her thoughts and behaviour. However, here, the inner critic has been specifically planted by the violent man and is particularly vicious and undermining. Along similar lines, Anjali described herself as 'broken and I can't be fixed', and talked about 'being conditioned' by her ex-partner 'to think that I am so awful':

> I am broken and I can't be fixed. The physical pain in my fingers [from an injury incurred during domestic violence] is especially bad, but the psychological damage is much, much worse. After years of being conditioned by him to think that I am so awful, it's really hard to retrain those voices in my head that are constantly repeating the same words he said to me over and over again. I am very damaged and don't trust people and tend to keep to myself more. I am not the happy go lucky person any more, I'm not smart anymore, I can't talk to people any more, I miss the old me very much. I am just the shell of the person I once was.
>
> (Anjali)

While Anjali's account describes the impact of the brain-washing techniques used by her partner, she also spoke with feeling about the grief of losing herself, captured in 'I'm not smart anymore, I can't talk to people anymore, I miss the old me very much'. In the next account, Veronica described how her partner's efforts to scapegoat and blame her were at first resisted but, over time, she began to question herself and think 'maybe I really am a bad person':

> Just feeling generally crap about yourself because you've stupidly chosen the wrong person so that, there's games that he played about twisting everything so it was my fault. You sort of take that on face value for a while and you question but you sort of think I guess I could've done it, you sort of rationalise it but then you start to 'think god, maybe I am a really bad person' ... and it is I'm still working my way through that.
>
> (Veronica)

Not dissimilarly, Freya said:

> They beat you down in a way in which you think you can't socialise with people, and they tell you you're doing everything wrong, and it takes a long while to learn how to talk to people again ... they beat you down to nothing and then it makes it hard to get jobs, makes it hard to talk to people, makes it hard to feel good about yourself, and it takes a long time to get that back.
>
> (Freya)

Here, Freya described the process of violence and coercive control as one of 'beating you down to nothing' until she believed she was both 'nothing' and 'wrong'. Again, this involves fracturing a woman's ontological security so that agentic action is difficult or even impossible. As this account shows, this sense of nothing-ness and wrong-ness is then directly linked to a lost sense of agency because it becomes difficult to act, including to interrelate with others and to obtain the basic necessities of life, such as employment. Felicia talked not dissimilarly about being 'worn down' to the point that she started to believe her partner's claim that she deserved nothing better:

> He actually wore me down to the point where I believed if I left him I wouldn't get anything better. That I, you know I should be thankful for everything he does for me because that's what I deserved and yeah, you actually, they wear your self-esteem down.... They make you feel like you need them, you can't survive without them.
>
> (Felicia)

The erosion of Felicia's agency and resistance led to feelings of worthlessness and an enforced dependence where 'you feel like you need them, you can't survive without them'. In addition to replaying a partner's abusive and denigrating words, the women's accounts capture the sheer oppression of coercive control, encapsulated in the analogy of being 'worn down', a term also used by Humphreys and Thiara (2003) to describe the impact of violence and control on women. Taking this further, while some women mentioned flashbacks and nightmares filled with fears of being killed or physically maimed, Lizzie described nightmares about her partner's oppression of herself and her children:

> There were some terrible nightmares about things and they were bizarre, like they weren't necessarily him being violent towards us but the oppression ... some of them were just he was doing really weird stuff that was oppressing us in other ways in the nightmares and things like maybe attacking me at work or – and it was to do with money and all sorts of really weird, weird nightmares, but just the exhaustion I know was the worst. Absolute exhaustion.
>
> (Lizzie)

Lizzie went on to say:

> That confidence just was completely knocked out of me, the wind's been knocked out of me and I remember going to the very first counsellor and saying to her three years before I left my husband I feel like someone's sitting on my chest and I can't breathe. He was so controlling that when I'd come home at night he'd lock the door so I couldn't get in so I'd have to wake him and then he'd follow me around and ask me 40 questions. The control tactics were so oppressive that that's taken me a long time to get out of [it].
>
> (Lizzie)

Lizzie directly linked the oppression of coercive control to difficulties with maintaining a sense of identity during this period: she said, 'it was a really exhausting process, keeping, maintaining, getting to work but also maintaining a level of self-identity and it's taken me a long time to realise a lot of these things'. Focusing on Lizzie's symptoms, such as lost confidence, breathing difficulties, nightmares and exhaustion might point a health practitioner to a diagnosis of PTSD, however, this would obscure the gendered dimensions of her experience. Hence, it is not only the physical threat of violence that has caused Lizzie to feel the way she does: her partner's tactics of ownership and control of her *as a woman* are experienced as physically and emotionally suffocating, and she talked about becoming exhausted in the effort to retain some vestige of self-identity. Lizzie therefore described fighting to retain her identity in the face of her partner's efforts to extinguish it, showing how women might be experiencing symptoms of psychological and emotional distress but, at the same time, exercise agency.

In most of the above accounts, the women emphasised the impact of psychological abuse and coercive control on their sense of themselves, with the fear of physical violence often in the background to this. The following account from Vivien moves fear and the avoidance of serious injury and death to the foreground. In a different twist on lost sense of self, identity and agency, Vivien described a very distinctive process of virtually *becoming* her abusive partner in order to survive. Vivien's partner was violent and controlling to the point of sadism, and it was he who was earlier described as deciding to kill her when he realised she planned to leave him. He also exercised obsessive control over her day-to-day activities, where 'I was not allowed to do so much as a crossword [and] I was allowed nothing of my own'. Here, Vivien described her growing capacity to predict her partner's actions by feeling his feelings and, in effect, 'becoming him':

> I started to almost feel everything that he felt, to the point that he was like an angry volatile person [and] I remember that he went to do something with the lawn mower and picked up a spanner and it was the wrong size and suddenly I could just feel this feeling of rage myself and feel myself shaking in anger, because it was the wrong size, because that was his reaction.... It was almost like I'd become him ... I feel it's almost a bit like a moth that went too close the flame, that for my own safety I had to be so hyper-aware. I even look back now and there's things that I could know by his footsteps. I remember this feeling of relief one night just thinking 'oh, somebody's going to come stay here tonight with him. And the person was still down at the pub, and we were going to be driving down later'. I could tell by his footsteps that somebody was going to actually come to his place in an hour or so's time ... whether it was his faster footsteps or he was ... a sort of a bit happy or something ... [and] I'd only just sort of realised not long ago that it was probably not a really normal thing, and something I'd never even questioned, all these funny little abilities that you end up with. Yes, I feel I was always having to be so tuned in to him for [my] own safety that it almost came a bit too far, and that I felt his emotion too much.... I still remember the day when I ... went to make a coffee and dropped the milk all over the floor and burst out laughing, and suddenly it was this thing of 'that's *my* reaction, I've got rid of him'. So it was like an exorcism of him from my system.
>
> (Vivien)

While Vivien suggested that this capacity to feel her partner's feelings was 'probably not a really normal thing', emotions are known to be 'catchy' in the sense that a person can feel something simply because another person does (Probyn, 2005). More specifically, though, Vivien's heightened capacity to catch and feel her partner's feelings developed in the very specific circumstance of having to be hyper-aware in a fundamentally unequal and dangerous power rela-tion. Thus, she presented extreme hypervigilance as leading to intuition, or a virtual sixth sense, in being able to predict what might happen next as if her partner was inside her: indeed, she told how she later 'exorcised' him from her system. While this phenomenon of feeling 'possessed' by her partner meant that Vivien was deprived to some extent of her own feelings about, and reactions to, events, 'becoming him' was an important survival mechanism that arguably enhanced agency by helping her act self-protectively in the face of threat. Thus, rather than pathologising such a phenomenon as dissociation that is symptomatic of PTSD, it might be better understood as an alternate form of agency in the face of gendered violence.

'Suddenly the world wasn't safe anymore': panic, agoraphobia and domestic violence

I now turn to examine women's explanations and experiences of panic and agoraphobia in response to violence and abuse as a further illustration of lost or changed sense of self and identity. A number of women in both the survey and the interviews mentioned experiencing panic and agoraphobia as a result of domestic violence and coercive control. While the general, less specific diagnosis of anxiety was the most commonly identified, I have chosen to explore in greater detail women's experiences of agoraphobia because it is a highly gendered diagnosis, an under-recognised consequence of gendered violence, it is especially debilitating in a day-to-day sense, and it specifically shows how fear in gendered violence can be pivotal to a lost sense of self and ontological insecurity. Agoraphobia is listed as an anxiety disorder in the DSM and commonly involves panic and anxiety in public spaces (APA, 2013). Panic attacks can then result in the individual feeling unable to leave the house because of fear that an attack will occur where there is no help or where symptoms might incur social embarrassment (APA, 2013). Over two-thirds of those diagnosed with agoraphobia are women (Davidson, 2000). Agoraphobia literally means 'a fear of open spaces', however, individual experiences are more complex than this and other spaces and situations can also be involved such that it is usually more about other people in the spaces in question than the spaces per se (Kirby, 1996, cited in Davidson, 2000). Within psychiatry, agoraphobia is understood to be related to 'neurotic disposition', negative childhood experiences such as poor attachment as a result of reduced parental warmth and over-protectiveness, and genetic vulnerability (APA, 2013). However, the DSM also acknowledges that 'being attacked' is a risk factor (APA, 2013: 220), although this is not elaborated and there is no mention of, or attempt to account for, gender differences in the presentation of agoraphobia. Nonetheless, evidence exists that agoraphobia is more common in women with histories of domestic violence compared to other women (Saunders, 1994), although there is little specific literature on this.

In the survey, 41.2 per cent of the women who reported a diagnosis of a mental illness indicated an anxiety disorder of some kind, with the question specifically listing PTSD, panic disorder and agoraphobia as examples. Thus, the women were not asked to specify which type of anxiety disorder they had been diagnosed with. The text-based answers to the open-ended question about the impact of domestic violence on psychological and emotional wellbeing yielded further insights into the nature of anxiety experienced by the women. Of the 557 women who answered this question, 26 (5 per cent) mentioned agoraphobia or symptoms consistent with it, 34 (6 per cent) mentioned panic attacks, and 44

(8 per cent) mentioned PTSD, which commonly includes symptoms of panic. Because the specific identification of agoraphobic symptoms by women in the survey was unprompted, it is likely that others had similar experiences but did not report them. The interviews revealed more in-depth insights into women's experiences of panic and agoraphobia, with five of the 17 women describing panic and the avoidance of public and other specific types of spaces. Hence, Vivien described feelings of panic and not being able to go to the shops; Sascha mentioned panic attacks and having difficulty going out; May described panic attacks, social phobia and agoraphobia to the point of not wanting to go out at all; Evelyn described panic attacks and not being able to leave the house by herself; and Veronica described panic attacks and developing fears about driving as a result. Some of the women experienced these symptoms while still with their violent partners, and others after they had left. No qualitative studies have specifically examined women's experiences of agoraphobia in contexts of domestic violence, and the following analysis therefore provides some new insights into this. The following extract from the survey responses provides an example of one woman's experience of agoraphobia:

> [Domestic violence] has impacted on my emotional wellbeing as I am afraid to leave my home. He also used family court to take my children from me even though he abused not only me but also the children.... Court is used as a weapon by him and it is a PTSD trigger ... last time no one believed or helped me and I now have a mistrust of police and judges. I have panic attacks when I leave the house. I have nightmares and I am very jumpy at every sound.
>
> (Daphne)

Here, panic and being afraid to leave the house are directly linked to both fear of violence but also to the partner's manipulation of the children and Daphne's distress about not being believed by powerful authority figures. Vivien provides some further insights into how she perceived the world as a result of domestic violence and coercive control, and how this linked to panic and agoraphobia. Vivien described violence and control as having opened a window onto a whole new world of fear that is completely outside the 'normal' world other people inhabit:

> I think the worst things about domestic violence is not, it's almost not what you think that it would be. It's that it's disorienting, that the world that you think you know, the normal everyday world, is suddenly completely different ... you'd be sitting in this unit thinking 'I'm a prisoner here', and you think the doors are unlocked, there's this normal street that I know there's the shops that I know so well down there, but I can't actually get out to them, it's as though, you know, it's as though he's got me locked in ... so it's not actually a fear at all, it's safety. And so to try to work out in your head which part's fear and which part is genuine danger is just impossible and all I wanted was somebody that could sit down in a balanced way and

say look you know, this is what it is ... because I remember spending some nights in the unit thinking about leaving him and I'd hear these noises and I'd think it would be him with a gun, and he'd have an unregistered gun and he did threaten to shoot me. And so you'd be saying to yourself, you know, look calm down, that's paranoid. And then you'd think of all these other things that were paranoid and stupid, and yet they'd actually happen. So all of a sudden you don't know what can happen and what can't happen. And so I ended up, you end up not quite living in the normal world, you just see this more frightening world.

(Vivien)

Vivien talked about 'sitting in this unit thinking "I'm a prisoner here" ... the doors are unlocked, there's this normal street that I know there's the shops that I know so well down there but I can't actually get out to them', because the world had come to feel inherently unsafe. However, she was confused about what was real and what was imagined, wanting someone to sit her down and tell her. After fleeing her violent partner, Vivien was placed in a block of public housing flats where there was serious conflict and violence between tenants, including threats of violence to her, contributing further to her sense of the world as unsafe. She went on to say 'I lost all sense of any normal safe world' and that 'at first, I was terrified of everyone, seeing every man as some sort of violent criminal', going on to say:

When I'd walk down the street, all I would see were like predators and victims and every time I got in the taxi I thought I was being driven to be murdered. And so even when I got out unscathed, I wouldn't think 'oh, well that was silly, or he wasn't a murderer', I'd think 'he's going to kill some- body different today, lucky it wasn't me today'.

Q: Those thoughts are quite intrusive, still now?
A: It wasn't thoughts ... when I talked to the psychologist, I said it's like there's two worlds and that I'm like today, I'm in the normal world ... so the one that you're in, [but] when a bit much happens, it's like flick- ing a switch [and when I am threatened or witness violence] I'm instantly in this other world and there's no concept of the normal world existing, all I see is this sort of horror.

(Vivien)

Vivien's account offers some very important insights into the impact of gendered violence on identity and one's sense of place in the world. First, she described the world of violence and abuse as peopled only by (male) predators and (female) victims, with herself in the powerless position of prey. Next, she insists to the inter- viewer that this perception 'wasn't thoughts ... there's two worlds'. Thus, Vivien described experiencing two different realities, with the violent world carrying all the feelings and perceptions wrought by gendered violence and coercive control as well as the day-to-day violence of the socially disadvantaged area in which she now lives. The movement between these two worlds was also described as instant and situational, and not related to particular thoughts, 'like flicking a switch'. This challenges the common assumption in cognitive psychology that an individual's feelings and perceptions are always caused, first and foremost, by specific and identifiable thoughts rather than by thought and feeling as one (Williams, 1977) or by a more direct perception of reality (Parker, 1992). Further to this, within cognitivist psychological theories, the 'normal everyday world' would be the correct and rational one while the world of violence and abuse would be the 'wrong' one, producing cognitive distortion and unwarranted feelings of panic and fear about going out in public: indeed, Vivien herself divided the two worlds in a similar way herself by calling the first world 'everyday' and 'normal' while the second is 'the other world'. While trauma theory might not insist on pre-existing irrational thoughts, it would nonetheless position Vivien's perception of the 'normal everyday world' becoming 'suddenly completely different' as symptomatic of trauma-related 'derealisation' rather than reflective of another lived, equally real and valid reality. As previously noted, in contrast to psychological theories such as these, Williams' (1977) concept of 'structures of feeling' theorises feeling and thought together as social rather than as privatised and individual experiences. Using such an understanding, Vivien's (and other women's) fear in 'the other world' reflects the correctly perceived, lived reality of gendered violence and abuse. Vivien had been diagnosed with PTSD and, while she did not particularly question this, the diagnosis seemed completely unequal to her dynamic explanation of panic in agoraphobia and its basis in a gendered social reality. Many other women also mentioned being diagnosed with PTSD, or embraced the diagnosis for themselves, and this seemed to be because it at least recognised that their distress emanated from violence and abuse rather than from their own individual psychopathology. I explore this further in the next chapter.

Not dissimilarly to Vivien, May talked about discovering an unsafe world through violence and abuse: 'suddenly the world wasn't safe anymore and I thought "I'm five foot two, how do I defend my kids?" This is not fair, it's totally unjust'. Again, May alludes to power inequalities when she emphasises her physical size and reduced capacity to protect herself because she cares for dependent children, relative to her partner's greater size and relative freedom. She went on to describe how long-term her sense of this unsafe world was:

Once he left town that [anxiety] lifted. But there was always – I remember him looking at me one day and saying 'You just make sure you keep looking over your shoulder – you won't know when it's coming'. And he said that years after we had broken up and it was like on my mind quite a bit.

Q: What effect did that have saying that?
A: Oh well again the world's not safe – check, check, check – didn't help my anxiety levels but at the same time I thought if I just sit around in the house he's won.

(May)

May expressed a strong sense of the injustice of living in an unsafe world where only she can keep herself and her children safe by checking and looking over her shoulder. Other women in the survey also mentioned learning that the world is an unsafe place because of domestic violence and feeling frightened outside the house as a result. For example, Patty said:

> I endure flashbacks, I am often teary. I believe I will never get free of the perpetrator.... I don't like being outside in my garden as I feel unsafe. I often feel angry.... I feel fearful a lot of the time. I see the world as an unsafe place and I am always waiting for when my ability to control my life will be impacted on again.
>
> (Patty)

Diagnosis of agoraphobia among women escalated in the 1950s and 1960s during a powerful reassertion of a domestic and dependent femininity in the post-war era when women were encouraged out of the workforce, where they had undertaken 'men's' work during the war, and into the home as home-makers, wives and mothers (Bordo, 1989). In line with this, Bordo (1989) has theorised agoraphobia as an exaggeration of femininity – as both a capitulation to gender oppression but also as protest – that is – 'You want me in the home? You shall have me in the home – with a vengeance!' (Bordo, 1989: 17). Domestic violence and coercive control involve an attempt to entrap women in the home and a traditional femininity in one of the most extreme ways possible, and women's refusal to leave the house as a result could be understood to signify, at a broad and metaphorical level, both a capitulation to the dictates of gendered violence and a protest against it. However, this plays down the severe nature of panic and fear in agoraphobia, whereby women commonly feel as if they simply *cannot* leave the house or enter certain spaces: as Vivien said of staying within her flat, 'I'm a prisoner here'. This undermines to some extent the idea of agoraphobia as protest by drawing attention to women's feelings of intense fear and powerlessness in such situations. Davidson's (2000) qualitative feminist study of women's experiences of agoraphobia in the UK shows how debilitating and frightening panic in agoraphobia can be. She demonstrates how panic is often experienced as stripping away the individual's sense of identity so that the outside world feels as if it is 'tearing in' on them and she argues that 'the felt boundary of the body has broken down' in this situation (Davidson, 2000: 33–34). Thus, as Davidson (2000) suggests, panic specifically involves a deep sense of ontological insecurity for the individual and retreating into the home can re-create the lost boundaries of the self through the four walls of the house, providing what Bordo (1989) has described as 'the foundation of an ontologically secure existence' (p. 90). There is an awful irony, though, in women who have experienced gendered violence feeling safest in the very place they have usually been most attacked and oppressed: as Patty said, 'I feel safe in spaces where I probably shouldn't because the most unsafe place for me was in my home'. However, the gendered identities of women are still more likely to be tied up with the home and the domestic realm than those of men, and women's retreat into this space might be therefore understood as a retreat into a more feminised space where they feel bounded and safe (Davidson, 2000).

For some women, though, fear and panic in certain spaces was more specifically related to their awareness of being at real, increased risk of violent attack by ex-partners in some places more than others. Others felt specifically unsafe in their *homes* as part of violence-related agoraphobia. For example, Kirsten and Patty said:

I suffered severe agoraphobia and depression during the years of abuse. I suffered panic attacks when I was subjected to abuse which incited more abuse. I have been diagnosed with post-traumatic stress disorder after several attempts on my life by my abusive partner towards the end of the relationship. I still have very low self-esteem and issues with trust and close relationships. I am still fearful of my partner and frequently wake with bad dreams or feel unsafe in my own home.

(Kirsten)

I often don't feel safe in my own home, it takes huge amounts of energy to function every day.... I feel fearful a lot of the time. I see the world as an unsafe place and always waiting for when my ability to control my life will be impacted on again.

(Patty)

In contrast, other women placed the emphasis on fear of being alone rather than fear of specific places, reflecting Kirby's point that agoraphobia is often more about the people in certain spaces rather than the spaces per se (Kirby, 1996, cited in Davidson, 2000). Thus, the function and meaning of home and public space differed depending on the nature of the violence women had faced, as did the function and meaning of symptoms of panic, fear and agoraphobia. Nonetheless, whether anxiety and panic revolved around public spaces, home or simply being alone, these experiences were connected by fear and the women's sense of lost sense of self, ontological insecurity and vulnerability in a world they have come to experience as inherently unsafe.

Gendered violence, conflicted identities and mental health

This analysis has demonstrated that lost sense of self and changed self-identity are central to many women's understandings and experiences of the impact of gendered violence and coercive control on their mental health. As the above analysis shows, the women's narratives include lost sense of self borne of the need to interpret and defer to the wishes of their partners, lost sense of self or the development of a negative self-identity in response to verbal denigration, and lost sense of self related to fear and panic in a world that has come to feel unsafe because of physical violence and coercive control. The women's accounts also foregrounded certain emotions as part of this, including feelings of low self-esteem, confusion, worthlessness, fear, shame and guilt, sadness, feeling wrong, stupid and powerless, feelings of grief at the loss of the old self, and feeling numb and empty. However, many women also expressed shock and anger at being deprived of their sense of themselves through male-perpetrated violence and control, reflecting the slippage between many contemporary women's expectations of love and a level of gender equality from male partners against the lived realities of violence, coercive control and denigration. Thus, the women's narratives captured diverse and conflicted feelings which were linked to an ontological insecurity in terms of lost sense of self, identity and agency.

As noted in earlier chapters, psychological trauma theorisations also centre the idea of lost sense of self and identity as a result of violence and abuse. Trauma theory suggests that abuse causes or exacerbates a deficient sense of self and self-identity, although there is rarely any mention of anger and resentment towards abusive men in the list of symptoms. As noted earlier, at this point in time, PTSD is one of the most common diagnoses given to women with these symptoms. Even though trauma theory and PTSD acknowledges the role of traumatising events, psychological theorisations are underpinned by a deficit understanding where the traumatised individual is nonetheless considered dysfunctional against the 'healthy norm' of the sufficiently bounded individual with strong, continuous identity and self-esteem. However, the women's accounts were largely devoid of such self-pathologisations and, as in other studies (Humphreys and Thiara, 2003), instead drew a direct causal link between the abuse and their feelings about themselves and the world. Moreover, while fear brought on by physical violence is central to notions of 'trauma' and PTSD, and many women described experiencing intense fear at times, it was the dehumanisation and depowerment of coercive control that received the greatest attention in their narratives. However, even though the women tended not to pathologise themselves in the way of psychology and medicine, they nonetheless depicted themselves as subject to *lesser* identities as a result of gendered violence and abuse. Next, I turn to examine the gendered assumptions and discourses about Western ideals of selfhood on which this construction was predicated.

In Western culture, the self is assumed to be autonomous, bounded and agentic with a stable, continuous identity over time (Rose, 1996). This is the very basis of the Western ideal of individual selfhood and it is this generic notion of self that the women evoked when they described themselves as lost or changed because of domestic violence and coercive control. Thus, the women's narratives relied on Western humanistic discourses of selfhood to portray gendered violence as robbing them of their basic human entitlements to autonomy and choice, leaving them to embody socially inferior identities that were sometimes experienced as involving no identity or self at all. Wirth-Cauchon (2001) suggests that psychiatrists and other clinicians have increasingly observed since the 1970s an increase in the numbers of patients describing uncertainty of identity. She argues that there has been a 'shift in vocabulary towards self and the appearance of crises of selfhood' that is 'part of a wider proliferation of discourses and practices of selfhood'

(Wirth-Cauchon, 2001: 14). Drawing on Foucault and other post-modern social theorists, Nikolas Rose (1996) has called this growing focus on the self 'the regime of the self', and he argues that the 'psy' disciplines of psychology and medicine are central to this, perpetuating a 'regulative ideal' of the self as inhabited by 'an inner psychology that animates and explains our conduct and strives for self-realisation, self-esteem, and self-fulfilment in everyday life' (Rose, 1996: 3). Wirth-Cauchon (2001) argues that this then becomes 'the regulative norm against which unstable selves are measured' (p. 15).

Feminists have long questioned the neutrality and universality of the Western ideal of the autonomous, bounded self. Theorists such as Butler, Clément, Irigaray and Beavoir have shown how this conception is conflated with conceptions of masculine subjectivity where women are constructed as 'other', 'overdetermined by the feminine position in the gender binaries of patriarchal logic' (Wirth-Cauchon, 2001: 84). More specifically, as Showalter attests, 'feminist theorists have shown how women, within our dualistic systems of language and representation, are typically situated on the side of irrationality, silence, nature, and body, while men are situated on the side of reason, discourse, culture and mind' (Showalter, 1987: 4). Thus, feminists argue that women's identity in this binary logic has been unstable and marked by paradox, contradiction, ambiguity and confusion, with women finding themselves in a representational and material double-bind between the idea of the traditional, essential feminine and the supposedly gender-neutral norm of ideal of healthy, normal selfhood as defined by psychology (Wirth-Cauchon, 2001).

In her analysis of women's location on the borderlines of subjectivity in the highly gendered diagnostic category of 'borderline personality disorder', Wirth-Cauchon (2001) elaborates further on critical feminist thought about the double-bind of subjecthood for women in Western cultures, and the implications for understanding women's struggles in relation to mental health and illness. She draws on the French feminist theorist Clément's (1986) notion of 'the interstices' as the spaces occupied by those with a dangerous symbolic mobility. Like other well-known post-structural feminists such as Butler (1990) and Irigaray (1985), Clément (1986) draws on Levi-Strauss's analysis of women's position in the sex-gender system as an object of exchange in patriarchal culture and yet as an anomaly in the interstices of the cultural order, that is, women are understood as double, on the boundaries between nature and culture (Clément, 1986, cited in Wirth-Cauchon, 2001). According to Levi-Strauss (1969, cited in Wirth-Cauchon, 2001), in cultures such as our own that are built on gift exchange, women have historically had the status of a gift exchanged in marriage by their fathers, and not that of a subject who exchanges. Women are therefore 'located in the interstices of social exchange, off-centre from subjecthood, serving the medium of exchange between subjects' (Wirth-Cauchon, 2001: 81) but without an identity of their own. Also drawing on the ideas of Beauvoir (1989), Wirth-Cauchon (2001) points out that 'woman' is also defined as 'lack' because 'in the logic of the gender binary, the category of "woman" is positioned as Other, a lack against which the masculine subject defines itself' and that the universal (male) subject therefore garners its meaning through the exclusion and repression of the feminine (Beauvoir, 1989, cited in Wirth-Cauchon, 2001: 84). Thus, feminists have argued that 'the place of woman is inhabited by the devalued projections of Western masculinist culture' (Wirth-Cauchon, 2001: 85). Importantly, though, 'woman' is also 'the sex', meaning she appears to men as an essentially sexual being (Beauvoir, 1989). Wirth-Cauchon (2001) points out that women are not simply exchange objects (or 'lack' or 'sex'), though, because even in a patriarchal man's world, a woman is still a person. This, then, is the basis of the double-bind of femininity – women are both subject and object.

Early second wave feminist work on domestic violence certainly pointed out that women were often viewed and treated as property rather than persons by violent and controlling men. However, the diverse socio-historical dimensions and drivers of such practices, their relation to patriarchal structures, and the implications for women's subjectivities and mental wellbeing have not been explicitly drawn out. In an effort to theorise these connections, I argue that the women's narratives of lost sense of self and identity closely mirror their positioning as 'objects of exchange' in violent and controlling relationships. I also argue that lost sense of self, identity and self-esteem are a manifestation of the devaluation of femininity that is so central to coercive control. First, descriptions of some of the tactics of coercive control position the women as sexualised 'objects' rather than as subjects in their own right. Practices such as monitoring and restricting the women's sexual behaviour and clothing are concerned with securing ownership over the women from other men, while rape is a specific way of reinstating property rights over the women's bodies in the face of (usually imagined) incursions from other men. Other practices such as taking control of earnings and enforcing domestic chores also position the women as property and as servicers of the men's needs rather than as persons or subjects in their own right. Thus, some of the tactics of coercive control appear to enact historical gender discourses and practices that position women as sexualised objects of exchange who service male identities but have little or no status or power as subjects with identities themselves. Moreover, in line with Stark's (2007) observations, such tactics appear to escalate when women act autonomously, as if the identities of violent and controlling men are reliant on female dependence and threatened by female independence.

Second, some of the tactics of violence and control described by the women involved a specific and targeted attack on femininity, suggesting that in gendered violence in particular, masculine identity relies on difference from, and devaluation of, femininity. Indeed, Stark (2007) offers evidence that violent men define their own attitudes and views as reasonable, rational and correct while the feminine is taken to be representative of the emotional, irrational and immoral. Further to this, though, Anderson (2009) argues that this masculine identity is a fragile one because, as humans, controlling men experience the very qualities they deny and seek to project onto women. Some of the women's depictions of verbal denigration seem to demonstrate a debasement of femininity that may well be fuelled by processes of projection and the establishment of difference.

Hence, some women described being denigrated for being stupid, mad, bad (for example, for imagined 'sexual promiscuity'), dependent (including when the male partner was in fact the dependent party), and they were specifically scapegoated and blamed for the men's own abusive behaviour. As noted earlier, these forms of abuse draw on a host of gendered femininity discourses that rest on the binary logic of the rational, controlled, autonomous and moral masculine and the irrational, emotional, dependent and immoral feminine. Again, this locates women as 'non-persons' against the rational masculine subject. The women also described being specifically controlled and criticised about housework and childcare duties. These tactics were more expressly concerned with attacking stereotypically feminine areas of responsibility and, as such, they drive at the heart of important areas of feminine identity, agency and self-esteem for women. Other research undertaken by myself and my colleagues demonstrates that these areas of feminine agency, particularly mothering, are critically important to positive identities for many women, and that refusing to leave violent relationships is not uncommonly bound up with efforts to meet mothering and homemaking expectations in the socially idealised and preferred structure of the two-parent family (Moulding *et al.*, 2015). Taken together, then, the women's reduction to object status alongside a denigration of 'feminine' qualities and responsibilities is powerful because it locates them as both 'non-persons' *and* as 'failed women'. This draws attention to the peculiarly gendered dimensions of lost sense of self, identity and agency in the context of domestic violence and coercive control.

Where women may have had much less opportunity in the past to resist a positioning as non-persons or attacks on feminised areas of identity, it seems at this historical juncture that many women will experience these depowered positions as fundamentally at odds with their sense of themselves *as* selves with rights and identities in line with other contemporary discourses of the individual. This is not to suggest that women who experience themselves as changed by violence and control have never been positioned in these ways before: all women in patriarchal societies are subjected to some extent to gendered cultural discourses and practices that undermine female personhood. Rather, as for child sexual and emotional abuse, I argue that gendered violence and coercive control involve a more extreme permutation of these, revealing the subject contradictions of contemporary femininity that might otherwise remain hidden or at least somewhat obscured. However, women with prior histories of gendered abuse and mental health problems have already been exposed in extreme ways to such contradictions, which are then re-experienced through domestic violence and coercive control, potentially enhancing their impact even further. Thus, women who experience domestic violence and coercive control encounter particularly conflicted, emotion-charged gender subject positions that exemplify and exaggerate more general contradictions about femininity in late modern societies in the context of shifts in women's social positions, opportunities and identities. Wirth-Cauchon (2001) suggests that as gender relations change and femininity and masculinity are redefined, 'boundaries between genders shift, creating areas of ambiguity' in both theory but also in material relations between the sexes that impact on 'people's everyday sense of themselves as gendered beings' (p. 7). She goes on to argue that the diagnosis of women with 'borderline personality disorder' reveals particularly well the 'cracks in the gender order' at this historical juncture in terms of women's contradictory positioning as subjects/persons and objects/non-persons (Wirth-Cauchon, 2001). I argue that women's narratives of lost sense of self and identity in the context of domestic violence and coercive control not dissimilarly expose these same fissures and while borderline personality disorder (BPD) reveals them in more dramatic terms, much higher numbers of women are affected by domestic violence and coercive control. The impact of these conflicts on women are then produced and reproduced in medical and psychological discourses as 'post-traumatic stress disorder', 'anxiety' and 'depression', pasting over the cracks in the gender order by maintaining a focus on what's wrong with women rather than the dynamics of contemporary gender relations. Moreover, I argue that psychological trauma theory, with its decontextualised and gender-neutral view of the individual, is probably unequal to the task of theorising these psychosocial complexities and their emotional impact in sufficiently meaningful ways.

Critical feminist analysis of women's understandings and experiences of mental health problems in contexts of domestic violence is a particularly important sub-field of feminist abuse studies. This is because, unlike other forms of gendered abuse which largely occur in childhood and adolescence, domestic violence is primarily meted out to adult women. As such, it is not so easy for the 'psy' disciplines to bring developmental personality theories to bear on formerly well-functioning adult women. This is particularly the case when large numbers of women identify themselves as strong and confident prior to the violent relationship, as occurred in this study. It is also difficult to ignore the fact that many of the symptoms reported by the women who experienced domestic violence echo very closely those reported by women who have experienced childhood emotional, sexual and physical abuse. However, the women who have experienced domestic violence and mental health problems were more inclined to express anger at the injustice of their treatment. It is probably easier for women who have left abusive partners who were supposed to love and support them to express such anger than it is for girls and adolescents abused in families they may be wholly or partially dependent on, or for women who were abused as children a long time ago. Women who were abused as children or adolescents are also likely to have had developmental psychological theories applied to them that are deeply pathologising, depowering and silencing. However, among the women in this study, anger about domestic violence was not only directed at abusive men, the male gender more broadly or the injustice of domestic violence, but also at family and friends who many women saw as failing to support them through their difficulties. There were other contextual dimensions to the women's narratives and experiences, such as loss of social status and poverty as a result of violence, that were also important to their mental health experiences. These will be considered further in the next chapter.

This chapter has explored the impact of gendered violence and coercive control on women's emotional wellbeing. It has shown that gendered violence and coercive control involve ongoing fears for women about physical danger *and* the navigation of deep-seated, gendered contradictions about who they are, their worth and their place in the world. The chapter has shown how violence and control can open a window on 'other' worlds of danger and fear that are little understood by those who sit outside such experiences, and are perhaps only more horror-inspiring for this. Most significantly, the chapter has demonstrated how gendered violence and coercive control exaggerate the already existing gender contradictions in women's day-to-day lives about being at once subject and object, person and non-person. While all women face such contradictions to some extent, gendered violence 'turns up the volume' and thereby turns up the associated emotional distress, which is then overlayed with fears of physical and sexual violence. While this chapter and previous chapters have focused on the psychological and emotional challenges women face as a result of gendered violence, the next chapter considers the narratives and experiences of recovery and approaches to challenging practices of community ignorance and denial of domestic violence and other forms of gendered abuse.

Note

1 The data on domestic violence and mental health was gathered as part of the following study: Franzway, S., Wendt, S., Moulding, N.T., Zufferey, C. and Chung, D.: 'Gendered violence and citizenship: the complex effects of intimate partner violence on mental health, housing and employment'. The study is funded by the Australian Research Council as a Discovery Project, No.: DP1130104437.

References

Almeida, R.V. and Durkin, T. (1999) The cultural context model: therapy for couples with domestic violence, *Journal of Marital and Family Therapy*, 25(3), pp. 313–324.

American Psychiatric Association (APA) (2013) *Diagnostic and Statistical Manual of Mental Disorders – DSM-5*. Arlington: APA.

Anderson, K.L. (2009) Gendering coercive control, *Violence Against Women*, 15, pp. 1444–1457.

Beauvoir, S. de (1989) *The Second Sex*. Translated by E.M. Parshley. New York: Vintage.

Bordo, S. (1989) The body and the reproduction of femininity: a feminist appropriation of Foucault. In A.M. Jaggar and S.R. Bordo (eds), *Gender/Body/Knowledge: Feminist Reconstructions of Being and Knowing*. New Brunswick: Rutgers University Press, pp. 13–34.

Buchanan, F., Wendt, S. and Moulding, N.T. (2014) Growing up with domestic violence: what does protectiveness mean? *Qualitative Social Work*, 14(3), pp. 399–415.

Butler, J. (1990) *Gender Trouble: Feminism and the Subversion of Identity*. New York: Routledge.

Chung, D. (2005) Violence, control, romance and gender equality: young women and heterosexual relationships, *Women's Studies International Forum*, 28(6), pp. 445–455.

Classen, C., Field, N., Koopman, C., Nevill-Manning, K. and Spiegel, D. (2001) Interpersonal problems and their relationship to sexual revictimization among women sexually abused in childhood, *Journal of Interpersonal Violence*, 16(6), pp. 495–509.

Clément, C. (1986) The guilty one. In H. Cixous and C. Clément, *The Newly Born Woman*. Translated by B. Wing. Minneapolis: University of Minnesota Press, pp. 1–62.

Davidson, J. (2000) '…the world was getting smaller': women, agoraphobia and bodily boundaries, *Area*, 32(1), pp. 31–40.

Davies, B. (1991) The concept of agency: a feminist poststructuralist analysis, *Social Analysis*, 30, pp. 42–53.

DeKeseredy, W.S. (2011) Feminist contributions to understanding woman abuse: myths, controversies, and realities, *Aggression and Violent Behavior*, 16, pp. 297–302.

Freyd, J.J. (1997) II: violations of power, adaptive blindness and betrayal trauma theory. *Feminism and Psychology*, 7(1), pp. 22–32.

Giddens, A. (1997) *Modernity and Self-Identity*. Cambridge: Polity Press.

Herman, J.L. (1997) *Trauma and Recovery*. New York: Basic Books.

Humphreys, C. and Thiara, R. (2003) Mental health and domestic violence: 'I call it symptoms of abuse', *British Journal of Social Work*, 33(2), pp. 209–226.

Irigaray, L. (1985) *The Speculum of the Other Woman*. Translated by G.C. Gill. Ithaca, NY: Cornell University Press.

Johnson, C.H. (2005) *Come with Daddy: Child Murder-Suicide after Family Breakdown*. Crawley: UWA Publishing.

Johnson, M.P. (2011) Gender and types of intimate partner violence: a response to an anti-feminist literature review, *Aggression and Violent Behaviour*, 16, pp. 289–296.

Johnson, M.P., Leone, J.M. and Xu, Y. (2014) Intimate terrorism and situational couple violence in general surveys: ex-spouses required, *Violence Against Women*, 20(2), pp. 186–207.

Kirby, K.M. (1996) *Indifferent Boundaries: Spatial Concepts of Human Subjectivity*. New York: Guilford Press.

Laing, L. and Toivonen, C. (2010) *Evaluation of the Domestic Violence and Mental Health Pilot Project*. Faculty of Education and Social Work, University of Sydney.

Lamanna, M. (1999) Living the postmodern dream: adolescent women's discourse on relationships, sexuality and reproduction, *Journal of Family Issues*, 20(2), pp. 181–217.

Levi-Strauss, C. (1969) *The Elementary Structures of Kinship*. Translated by J. Harle Bell, J.R. von Sturmer and R. Needham. Boston: Beacon Press.

Lister, R. (2007) Inclusive citizenship: realising the potential, *Citizenship Studies*, 11(1), pp. 49–61.

McNay, L. (2004) Situated intersubjectivity. In B. Marshall and A. Witz (eds), *Engendering the Social: Feminist Encounters with Sociological Theory*. Maidenhead: Open University Press, pp. 171–186.

Morris, A. (1999) Adding insult to injury, *Trouble & Strife*, 40, pp. 30–35.

Moulding, N.T., Buchanan, F. and Wendt, S. (2015) Untangling self-blame and mother-blame in women's and children's perspectives on maternal protectiveness in domestic violence: implications for practice, *Child Abuse Review*, published online 12 May 2015, DOI: 10.1002/car.2389.

Nicolaidis, C., Gregg, J., Galian, H., McFaralnd, B., Curry, M. and Gerrity, M. (2008) 'You always end up feeling like you're some hypochondriac': intimate partner violence survivors' experiences addressing depression and pain, *Journal of General Internal Medicine*, 23(8), pp. 1157–1163.

Parker, I. (1992) *Discourse Dynamics: Critical Analysis for Social and Individual Psychology*. London: Routledge.

Probyn, E. (2005) *Blush: Faces of Shame*. Minneapolis: University of Minnesota Press.

Rose, N. (1996) *Inventing Ourselves: Psychology, Power and Personhood*. Cambridge, MA: Cambridge University Press.

Saunders, D.G. (1994) Posttraumatic stress symptom profiles of battered women: a comparison of survivors in two settings, *Violence and Victims*, 9(1), pp. 31–44.

Scheffer Lindgren, M.S. and Renck, B. (2008) 'It is still so deep-seated, the fear': psychological stress reactions as consequences of intimate partner violence, *Journal of Psychiatric and Mental Health Nursing*, 15(3), pp. 219–228.

Sharpe, S. (2001) Going for it: young women face the future, *Feminism and Psychology*, 11(2), pp. 177–181.

Showalter, E. (1987) *The Female Malady: Women, Madness, and English Culture, 1830–1980*. New York: Pantheon Books.

Stark, E. (2007) *Coercive Control: How Men Trap Women in Personal Life*. Oxford: Oxford University Press.

Stark, E. (2012) Re-presenting battered women: coercive control and the defense of liberty, prepared for the conference *Violence Against Women: Complex Realities and New Issues in a Changing World*, Les Presses de l'Université du Québec.

Walby, S. (1990) *Theorizing Patriarchy*. Cambridge, MA: Blackwell Publishers.

Walby, S., Towers, J. and Francis, B. (2014) Mainstreaming domestic and gender-based violence into sociology and the criminology of violence, *The Sociological Review*, 62(S2), pp. 187–214.

Williams, R. (1977) *Marxism and Literature*. Oxford: Oxford University Press.

Wirth-Cauchon, J. (2001) *Borderline Personality Disorder: Symptoms and Stories*. Piscataway: Rutgers University Press.

7 Putting abuse in its place
Living well and challenging community denial

> I want to laugh more, dance in my own lounge room, eat chocolate and have a
> cup of tea while reading a book and other small achievements before I die.
>
> (A woman after leaving domestic violence)

The above quote demonstrates how simple life pleasures can be for women after
years of gendered violence and abuse. This chapter explores the different ways
women described overcoming the mental health effects of abuse in their day-to-day
lives. Individual experiences were diverse and, rather than attempt to document the
multiple strategies employed as part of individual recoveries, the chapter instead
focuses on how women narrate the overall processes of recovery in terms of shifts
in identity and sense of self, the place of formal treatment in recovery, and the significance of positive, non-conditional relationships. Across these three themes, I
continue to consider how gender frames individual narratives and experiences. Relationships were especially important in women's explanations of overcoming the
effects of abuse. This should come as no surprise given that the women largely saw
their mental health problems as emerging in the context of violent, controlling and
conditional relationships: perhaps logically, then, they also understood and experienced their recoveries taking place in the context of supportive, non-conditional
relationships. However, this theme was more complex in the case of domestic violence, in part because of the nature of this kind of gendered abuse. Most importantly,
the chapter examines the implications of the narratives and experiences presented
throughout this book for helping professionals, and specifically engages with the
scope for feminist-informed approaches both to one-on-one practice but also to preventive community-wide intervention, which is often overlooked in this area.

Narrating recovery

Where participants in the studies reported on in previous chapters considered
themselves to have recovered from mental health problems, their narratives often
included descriptions of the processes of recovery and healing. It is important to
point out that some individuals, both women and men, who saw themselves as
recovered had not necessarily consulted with helping professionals: thus,

recovery took place both with and without professional assistance. Here, I consider how the overall process of recovery was constructed, the discourses called upon and their gendered dimensions, in particular, how women constructed new identities for themselves that enabled them to live more satisfying lives in spite of abuse and mental health problems.

Narrative theorists and researchers have identified certain narrative styles that are commonly used by individuals to explain overcoming adversity in their lives, and these can provide insights into shifts in identities and sense of self. As noted in Chapter 4, narratives of abuse often have a redemptive quality to them whereby the painful event is 'redeemed, salvaged, mitigated, or made better in light of the ensuing good' (McAdams *et al.*, 2001: 474, cited in Thomas and Hall, 2008). Similar to the redemptive narrative is the quest narrative, which is common in accounts of illness (Frank, 1995: 128). In this style of narrative, illness or adversity is presented as a major personal challenge that requires the individual to be 'more than she has been' (Frank, 1995: 128). The styles drawn on by the participants in my studies included redemptive and quest narratives. However, the use of certain narrative styles varied according to the type of abuse experienced, the type of mental health problem confronted and, related to this, to the gender discourses and practices in operation. As demonstrated in Chapter 4, some of the men's narratives about childhood emotional abuse focused around ideas of 'vanquishing the father' and becoming 'a better man', and these clearly involved redemptive and quest themes with significant gender dimensions. Because I have explored these in some detail already, I will not revisit them here other than to say that they enabled the men to construct themselves as 'good men', in control of their lives and guides to others. Paul's narrative also included acceptance that he would experience some level of anxiety for the rest of his life because of abuse, but he nonetheless talked with satisfaction about his life and his achievements. This reflects current recovery discourses about mental health, which posit that recovery is primarily about living well and with hope, and contrasts with traditional medical notions of cure (Anthony, 1993; Bland *et al.*, 2015; Deegan, 1996). As such, then, recovery can take place in spite of the presence of symptoms (Deegan, 1996). A number of participants constructed their recoveries in this way. Paul and two of the other men also centred religion as part of their redemptive stories, and I have already shown how this worked together with hegemonic masculinities to reinforce positive identities.

A couple of the women who experienced childhood emotional abuse and went on to struggle with mental health problems also constructed their narratives through the idea that, in addition to pain and suffering, they had gained from their experiences. For example, Catherine said:

> Well, I've been through things, I've overcome them, on a scale of human experience it's probably not as bad as some people and I am still – I still have four limbs, I still have not all of my family but I am not a single person in the world. I still do have … my sister, I have her and I have an amazing group of friends and I've got an amazing support network if I need it.
>
> (Catherine)

Catherine talked about becoming 'the person I am sort of meant to be' by going to university and doing volunteer work in the community. She described having dreams for herself now, and wanting to be active in human rights and political activism in spite of still sometimes struggling with panic disorder, again in line with contemporary recovery discourses. However, few of the women talked about turning to mainstream religion to overcome the effects of abuse. While Melissa grew up in an evangelical Christian family, she nonetheless rejected mainstream Christianity because of its traditional approach to gender, and talked about developing her own relationship with her version of god. Most organised religions are patriarchal institutions with conservative views and practices in relation to gender (Hajjar, 2004), so perhaps they might seem more useful to men in distress than to women. Redemptive themes in the women's narratives of childhood emotional abuse were also generally less clear-cut than in the men's. Perhaps this was in part because the women told of struggling with abuse for much longer, sometimes until they ended relationships with their abusers well into adulthood, and also because their narratives involved high levels of contradiction. Hegemonic masculinities may also tend to produce a more redemptive style of narrative through the idea of vanquishing and prevailing over abusers and abuse, while femininity discourses often ascribe a level of blame and guilt to women themselves.

The women who experienced childhood abuse followed by an eating disorder often presented their experiences as personal quests with redemptive themes, drawing on the metaphor of 'the eating disorder journey' (see Moulding, 2015, for a more detailed analysis of this). Along these lines, Rebecca described walking out of treatment for bulimia because her abuse was not acknowledged by her psychiatrist, and went on to present her recovery as a 'healing journey' that enabled her to develop a new pathway in life as a 'self-healer':

> I worked consciously with yoga and meditation over a period of, probably a year, and then it all [the bulimia] just stopped.... I've had to take an alternative path.... So, in the end it sort of propelled me on this path of self-sufficiency in being able to heal myself, knowing the avenues that I needed to take, and knowing what I could do to heal myself.
>
> (Rebecca)

Carole described her recovery process as one involving major self-transformation that included a deeper understanding of life:

> I don't regret my eating disorder, as funny as it sounds because it's made me the person I am. It's really opened my eyes to, I believe, what life is about, and I just learnt so much from it, and I don't regret it.
>
> Q: You feel like you've actually gained in the end?
> A: Yeah, in the end, yeah, yeah I do.... We all learn in ways, and that was my way of learning.
>
> (Carole)

By portraying the eating disorder as 'my way of learning', it becomes almost inevitable and something from which Carole ultimately benefited. This kind of narrative is also called 'auto-mythological' because it has strong themes of destiny (Frank, 1995). Carole went on to say:

> I wanted that tablet to cure me, and I wanted that counsellor to cure me. And then I realized they couldn't cure me, that there was no magic pill, that I had to do this, and I was the only one that had the ability to do this ... I had to accept and change my thought patterns or I was going to be unwell for the rest of my life.... You have to take that responsibility and make that decision, whether you want to be a victim in life and suffer.
>
> (Carole)

Thus, like Rebecca, Carole positioned herself as having overcome the eating disorder herself. As noted earlier, the approaches to recovery from the women who had experienced eating disorders were more reflective of traditional medical discourses that understand recovery as a relatively complete restoration of previous functioning (Davidson *et al.*, 2005) rather than of contemporary recovery discourses. Other qualitative studies have similarly emphasised the unique nature of recovery from an eating disorder compared to other mental health problems, where the disorder seems to become no longer part of a woman's life (Lamoureux and Bortorff, 2005; Bjork and Ahlstrom, 2008). This feature of recovering from an eating disorder might lend itself to a quest style of narrative: women have usually engaged in a significant struggle with themselves to overcome the drive for thinness and the use of food to manage negative emotion (Patching and Lawler, 2009). In line with this, many women spoke of having vanquished the disorder, with Rebecca in particular claiming 'I licked it! I cured myself!' Some women also presented themselves as putting a stop to emotional abuse in their day-to-day lives as part of their full recoveries. Thus, Rebecca said:

> I continued to battle this low self-esteem and I said [to my parents], 'you have to change the way you relate to me, otherwise I'm out of here and you will never see me again'. And they changed, they started changing. I became more empowered. I learnt about saying 'stop, OK, this is how I am feeling, and you are actually treating me in a disrespectful way and I am not going to allow you to do this to me anymore'.
>
> (Rebecca)

This contrasts with Rebecca's descriptions of having tried to please her parents in the past. Carole talked about ending her relationship with her mother as part of her full recovery:

> The way she'd been with me as a teenager, the spitefulness and that dangling her affection, she actually [started doing that] to my daughter. I could see she was, and that was what basically sort of cut the cord with me ... and

I just said to her, 'No more' ... and that was it, there's been no contact since.... And it's helped me immensely, cutting her out of my life.

(Carole)

Carole presented herself as actively putting a stop to behaviour she saw as abusive, powerfully captured in the statement, 'no more'. Thus, some of the women portrayed the eating disorder as having played an important role in making them the agentic individuals they now believe themselves to be, with religion also largely absent from these accounts but contemporary 'New Age' discourses about spirituality and self-healing important, instead (see also Garrett, 1998). While a valorisation of individual agency was therefore significant in some of these narratives, what also emerged as central was the place of positive, less gendered social relationships in helping the women forge these more positive, self-affirming identities and this is explored further later.

Narratives with redemptive or quest themes and structures were far less in evidence from the women who had experienced domestic violence. This in part reflects differences between the studies, with the first two specifically enquiring into recovery while the domestic violence study was more concerned with documenting the impact of violence on women's lives in relation to mental health, housing and employment. However, the lack of redemptive or quest themes among these women also reflects the nature of domestic violence itself and its impact on women's lives. Thus, while there were some examples of women who described becoming more assertive and caring of themselves because of violence and abuse, this was against the backdrop of the negative consequences of domestic violence not only on mental health but also on the material conditions of their lives in terms of housing, employment, income and social networks, which seemed to compound poor mental health for some women. Further to this, though, many women also described significant levels of social abuse as part of domestic violence, with violent men portrayed as purposely severing their access to support, and with community denial of, and blame for, domestic violence described as working to further isolate them. It is well-recognised that social isolation worsens mental health (Bland *et al.*, 2015), so this feature of domestic violence is likely to complicate women's capacity to overcome the effects of domestic violence. Another obvious difference between the women who had experienced partner violence and those who had experienced childhood abuse is that the abuse was much more recent for the former group, and many women had the additional challenge of caring for dependent children while they tried to manage the fall-out. Thus, most women were in no position to be considering any personal gains that may have flowed from confronting domestic violence and they mainly identified significant losses, instead, as well as the ongoing challenge of trying to manage their day-to-day lives. Thomas and Hall (2008) draw on McAdams *et al.* (2001) to define 'contamination' narratives as those where a 'good experience' is 'spoiled, ruined, contaminated, or undermined by what follows it' (McAdams *et al.*, 2001: 474, cited in Thomas and Hall, 2008: 150). It is somewhat trite to describe leaving domestic violence as a 'good experience' because the risks to women's and children's safety on leaving are so well-known, however, the additional problems described by many of the women in this study once they had left were sometimes so great that contamination themes were extremely common in their narratives. Along these lines, May said:

> I don't think I would be ill [but for domestic violence]. I don't think I would be sick. I don't think I would be on a pension. I just feel like [my life has] been stolen.... I've done my best but sometimes I feel like that's not enough but that's beside the point ... that's all I had to fight with. I had minimal tools. It was a case of survival.
>
> (May)

Lastly, because the women who had experienced domestic violence were adults when they were abused, many were able to comprehend the injustice of their treatment and expressed significant levels of anger about this: as noted in Chapter 6, anger was a discernible 'structure of feeling' among the women who had left domestic violence. Children may have little sense of their rights, and the process of coming to name their experiences as abuse and deal with the consequences therefore takes place over a long period of time as part of growing up and finding their way in the world: consideration of what also may have been learned from abuse is perhaps more likely in this context. Next, I consider participants' accounts of seeking formal help, with an eye towards what they found helped and what did not.

'It's not brain chemicals ... my life sucks': resisting medicalisation

Some individuals participating in the three studies did not seek professional help for their abuse-related mental health problems, although most women leaving domestic violence did. National Australian data reports that only 38 per cent of individuals in Australia with mental health problems access services (ABS, 2007). Of those who did seek help, there was great diversity in the type of services accessed, the extent to which they were found to be useful, and the reasons given for why they were not always beneficial. Many individuals sought help within the mainstream mental health and primary care systems. Not uncommonly, individuals consulted with general practitioners and some were then referred for counselling to social workers, psychologists, psychiatrists or other mental health counsellors. Those who experienced more extreme mental health problems received care in the tertiary mental health system, for example, through public and private psychiatric inpatient or out-patient units, while some of the women who experienced eating disorders received treatment in specialist public or private eating disorder units.

Across all of the studies, there were individuals who said that they had benefited from mainstream psychological treatments such as medication or various forms of interpersonal psychotherapy. However, there were also significant numbers who said that they did not find mainstream treatment useful. The reasons given varied across the studies, though. Hence, among those with histories of childhood emotional abuse, while fewer sought formal help than individuals in the other studies, a failure by professionals to connect their struggles with their histories of abuse was identified by some as problematic. Among the women with eating disorders, a one-size-fits-all approach to treatment, feeling misunderstood by practitioners and lack of connection with treating staff were common, however, mention was also made of not having abuse connected to their eating problems. Experiences among the women who had backgrounds of domestic violence were very diverse, however, there was also a common theme about resistance to having mental health problems medicalised and not connected to domestic violence. Thus, there were individuals in all three studies who constructed their mental health problems as primarily caused by violence and abuse, and this discourse was matched by a level of resistance to medical discourses and practices that sought to locate mental illness primarily within them as individuals. A further important theme about treatment emerged across all three studies: that it was not the type of therapy per se that was necessarily of critical significance but a good interpersonal connection with the helping professional (Bland *et al.*, 2015), as well as being believed about abuse and feeling understood.

A number of the participants described not feeling understood or being dismissed by helping professionals. Melissa mentioned being dismissed by a doctor when she described her depression, and went on to describe her sense that 'I don't really connect with [my psychologist] – I don't feel like I am really dealing with my issues'. The treatment she receives is primarily cognitive-behavioural with a focus on challenging so-called cognitive distortions. For example, Melissa said that her fears about visiting her emotionally abusive family were dismissed as merely 'in my imagination'. This speaks to one of the greatest potential problems with cognitive-behavioural approaches to working with abused clients: the risk of re-casting client fears as irrational rather than as reasonable given a history of abuse. Melissa also went on to say that she found the research interview itself therapeutic and she was not the only participant to say so: many participants said they found being listened to in a non-judgemental way and having the chance to name their experiences as abuse helpful. This emphasises the importance of simple, empathic listening and understanding (Bland *et al.*, 2015), because I was careful not to take on a counselling role as the researcher. Not dissimilarly to Melissa, Rebecca specifically mentioned how there was no connection between herself and her psychiatrist during her treatment for bulimia:

> I couldn't get through to him. He just wouldn't listen to me. He wouldn't explain to my parents how the bulimia was connected with how they were treating me…. He didn't go into any of that, it was just like, well this is – it was just, like the clinical presentation of the eating disorder…. He didn't go into the emotional abuse, nothing. He didn't say anything to them, and I went out then, and I thought, I'm never coming back, and I never went back.
>
> (Rebecca)

Rebecca emphasised the psychiatrist's refusal to listen but also his failure to acknowledge the connection between her mental health problems and her background of abuse. She left formal treatment at this point and, as noted earlier, found a pathway to recovery through self-care practices of yoga and relaxation therapy. Mariana talked about how a counsellor missed the signs of domestic violence during couple counselling when she mentioned her fear of her partner, choosing instead to label her as 'passive-aggressive':

> I was thinking, maybe if we had gone to a proper counsellor, maybe that counsellor could have picked it up [and said] 'when you said you are afraid of your partner, oh something is wrong'. But anyway, then they said I was passive-aggressive. And so.... I'm facing, well, the violence and the hate, he really hates me, his family really hates me, his father assaulted me.
>
> (Mariana)

Ignorance about domestic violence can be based on the presumption that couples are operating on an essentially equal playing field, and that both are therefore contributing equally to the 'conflict' in the relationship. However, such assumptions can add to a woman's struggles by labelling, pathologising and blaming her in the process. These testimonies draw attention to the interpersonal dimensions of care and how deficits in this area can completely undermine the therapeutic process. Some participants made a more forthright critique of the pathologising tendencies of medical and psychological approaches and how they can render backgrounds of abuse invisible. Catherine, who had experienced childhood emotional abuse, talked about how the psychiatric label given to her completely ignored the context of her life:

> I did that [psychological test] and then [they] said that I was manic-depressive.
>
> Q: Did you accept that at the time?
> A: No.
> Q: Do you now?
> A: No ... between when I was 11 to 17 was the worst time of my life. Dad died, Mum just lost it completely, and then all this stuff happened at school, that diagnosis, I just – I didn't go to school for basically a whole term. I literally sat in a room in the dark.
>
> (Catherine)

The impact of a diagnosis of bipolar disorder in the context of the domestic chaos and emotional abuse that Catherine lived with was described as resulting in her retreating into social isolation and further depression. Catherine believed she had a particularly negative reaction to this specific diagnosis because her abusive mother had also been diagnosed as 'manic-depressive'. Catherine later determined for herself that she probably has generalised anxiety disorder, and she avoids doctors for fear of being wrongly labelled and treated. Paul described being treated with medication for some ten years following the development of major anxiety triggered by two workplace accidents. The connection between Paul's mental health problems and emotional and physical abuse from his father was only made by a psychologist towards the end of that period, and many of the symptoms he had come to exhibit were later determined to be side effects from the prescription drugs he had been on for years rather than symptoms of mental illness itself. In a tale of incredible fortitude and good fortune in the face of adversity, Paul told of how he took a drug overdose in a desperate cry for help, went into a coma, and how many of his symptoms had disappeared when he regained consciousness because of the inadvertent break from the prescription drugs. However, in a reversal of Paul's experience of medical misadventure, Vanessa told of 20 years of disappointing psychotherapy, marked by flickers of hope followed by crushing despair that she would never be free of the extreme panic that suddenly overcame her in her early twenties following years of child-hood sexual and emotional abuse. Vanessa described eventually finding an empathic psychiatrist who diagnosed her with PTSD, prescribed anti-anxiety drugs and how her life turned around from that point on.

The group of participants who were the most vocal and angry about medical-ised responses to their mental health problems were the women who had experi-enced domestic violence. However, like Vanessa above, some of these same women also embraced a diagnosis of PTSD, although many believed that treat-ment with medication was inappropriate for them. It is important to remember that the greater proportion of women in this group had no history of mental health problems prior to domestic violence, and this might partly explain their strong resistance to medicalised approaches to their distress. Amelia argued with some passion that her diagnosis of borderline personality disorder and bipolar disorder are not appropriate and that, instead, she is suffering from PTSD:

> The courts [are] trying to say I have a borderline personality disorder. 'Sorry lovie, I don't tick enough boxes for that one, I don't tick enough boxes for borderline'. And I've had four other psychs tell me the same shit, who knew nothing each time. I'm suffering post-traumatic stress disorder, and my ADHD [attention deficit hyperactivity disorder] aggravates it a lot, but I don't have borderline personality disorder and I don't have bipolar.
>
> (Amelia)

For Amelia, a diagnosis of BPD and of bipolar disorder are part of a campaign to discredit her as 'mad' and therefore an unfit mother. However, she considers a diagnosis of PTSD acceptable and appropriate. As noted earlier, unlike other psychiatric diagnoses, PTSD potentially acknowledges the role of gendered violence in women's distress and therefore places the causes outside the woman and in her situation. Gertrude said that while she was not formally diagnosed with PTSD, she suspects she has had it and that she still experiences some vestiges of it:

I was certainly not diagnosed with post-traumatic stress but I wouldn't be surprised if I suffered from it because I still have well even now I still have occasional nightmares about him trying to get to me.

(Gertrude)

May explained that she sought the help of a counsellor because even though her partner was raping her and threatening to kill her, her doctor only offered a tranquiliser. May went on to explain that her counsellor referred her to a psychiatrist and that it was he who diagnosed her with PTSD: she believes this diagnosis to be correct. PTSD gives May scope to understand and explain her distress as borne of gendered violence and not of some pre-existing quality or vulnerability within herself. Thus, for May, the diagnosis of PTSD can acknowledge the impact of gendered violence and coercive control on her life without pathologising her in an essentialist way. Nonetheless, PTSD still places women's violence-related distress within a medical framing. It also defines women's trauma as 'post' despite the fact that many who have experienced domestic violence remain in real danger for many years after they leave, unlike other individuals whose diagnosis of PTSD is related to discrete events. As Lizzie so poignantly said: 'you never really get away, unless they're dead, I suppose'. Even more concerning, though, is the propensity for a diagnosis of PTSD, or any psychiatric diagnosis for that matter, to obscure the gendered dimensions of violence and abuse. This is quite graphically illustrated in Vivien's description of the two worlds of abuse-related agoraphobia in the previous chapter. Having explained her perception of the 'normal' world and the 'other' world inhabited by predators and prey, the interviewer asked Camille what her psychologist made of this. Vivien answered that 'she said that it was a symptom of post-traumatic stress'. While Vivien neither overtly accepts or rejects this diagnosis, it nonetheless has the effect of flattening out her account so that the evocative and dynamic depiction of a world peopled only by (male) predators and (female) victims is effectively lost because it becomes nothing more than 'cognitive distortion' wrought by trauma. Thus, Vivien's perceptions and feelings are individualised and also overwritten by a single diagnosis that is also given to individuals who have not experienced the peculiarly gendered dynamics and consequences of gendered violence and abuse.

Mary and Jane offered more direct and global challenges to psychiatric labelling and assumptions about biological causes of mental health problems in contexts of domestic violence. Mary described being labelled with one diagnosis after another, and she critiqued psychiatry for its 'overlapping' symptoms and lack of delineation between the different conditions:

[The doctor] told me that I had ADHD and I should see a psychiatrist. So I went and saw a psychiatrist who diagnosed me with PTSD as well. And then after we split up I saw a psychologist because I wasn't coping with it, and he told me he thought I had bipolar, so I saw another psychiatrist because mine retired. And he said that, yeah, it looked like I was bipolar.

But the one I'm seeing now said that I'm not actually bipolar, I'm just a kid with a lot of issues....

Q: So how do you feel about being given all those diagnosis, do they make sense to you?

A: The problem is they've all got overlapping symptoms and a lot of things can be environmental, because I haven't displayed any symptoms of bipolar for about a year now. So I think in times of stress I kind of go a little bit crazy and it looks like bipolar, but yeah.

Q: Maybe it's normal response to trauma?

A: Yeah.... That's what the current psychiatrist is thinking, yeah.

(Mary)

Mary concluded that her distress is environmental, and her current psychiatrist agrees, but this comes after significant labelling with conditions that are both serious and deeply pathologising. Jane made the compelling comment that 'the issue isn't the chemicals in my brain, the issue is my life sucks':

All GPs will do is just put you on antidepressants which don't work. The issue isn't the chemicals in my brain. The issue is my life sucks ... circumstantial depression isn't best treated by anti-depressants, anti-depressants are for ... stabilisation for chemical imbalances, it's not the right treatment, but it's all a GP can offer.

(Jane)

Jane described her depression as 'circumstantial' rather than related to brain chemicals. Lizzie was not dissimilarly critical of an emphasis on the use of medication when women are experiencing gendered violence and coercive control:

A couple of years before I left my husband I remember going to the GP and – my ex was being an absolute bugger ... it was one of those really bad patches and she offered me anti-depressants, in fact gave them to me there and then.... I was very nervous of taking them so I took them back a couple of months later and I said 'look it was a really bad patch, I just think I was struggling at the time with [my partner] not being there for me and him attacking me all the time'. And I actually gave them back to her and I said 'I want this on my record that I've given them back to you and I didn't take them' because I just didn't want it on my record.

(Lizzie)

Importantly, Lizzie wanted her medical record updated to show that she did not take the medication, meaning that she did not want the stigma of a psychiatric diagnosis and treatment to be documented. This is a powerful reminder that being given such a diagnosis involves accepting a socially devalued and pathologised identity. Lizzie said: 'I've got friends who have suffered from depression all their life. I get that they need the medication', but she was completely unwilling to accept that this explained her situation. Moreover, women are also aware that health records can be subpoenaed by ex-partners in custody battles to portray women as unfit mothers (see also Humphreys and Thiara, 2003), so psychiatric diagnosis can have particularly devastating consequences for women in contexts of gendered violence. Lizzie went on to talk about finding a counsellor who understood her distress as reflective of her situation, and who instead focused on her strengths in having managed in this context.

Relationships and recovery

The theme of social relationships and their contribution both to the development of mental health problems in the first place, and then to overcoming these problems later, was central across all of the studies. Clearly, the individuals in all the studies saw their mental health problems as largely stemming *from* their experiences in relationships, so the fact that the development of supportive, non-abusive relationships was portrayed as crucial to overcoming the effects of abuse is hardly surprising. Moreover, as noted, it is well-known that positive, supportive relationships are crucial to good mental health (Bland *et al.*, 2015).

Unconditional relationships

Among those who had experienced childhood emotional abuse, many individuals talked about the importance of finding other older individuals during childhood who could give them the unconditional love and support they were not receiving from their parents. Abusive relationships often involve high levels of conditionality, where victims are only valued in so far as they benefit their abuser in some way (Doyle, 2001), so it is unsurprising that it was non-conditional regard that was so highly valued by participants. Melissa talked about support from an older couple at her church:

> They were presbytery caretakers and they were lovely, they were ... really, really nice, and I didn't understand how like a male the same age as my dad could be so nice and just gentle.
>
> Q: He was such a contrast?
> A: Yeah a huge contrast and he kind of confused me a bit – at first I thought what's wrong with this person? A very, very calm person, very gentle and [it was] grand-parenting.
>
> (Melissa)

Catherine talked about her older sister, who she described as her 'mother-sister' and as having given her all the support and unconditional love that her parents could not.

> She just always – I know that we fought, and I know that things went bad for a
> little while. But I knew that I had unconditional love from one person. I knew
> that she was the only – her and [this other friend] were the only people that
> would love me unconditionally and – I felt though, as though I owed it to her
> [to go to university] because she had given up her education. I was like I can
> never do that. And even now, whenever I do – whenever I get an HD or I do
> really well, I'm like hey, guess what? And she's like…. She's so proud of me.
>
> (Catherine)

Significant support people were sometimes older sisters, brothers, neighbours,
teachers or caring people through a local church (see Doyle, 2001) and participants described being helped to see their potential and encouraged into studies or
other activities they were interested in by these supportive individuals. As also
found by Doyle (2001), though, this type of support was rarely found with the
non-abusive parent, if there was one, or from grandparents, perhaps reflecting
the levels of conflict and distress within and across generations in many of the
participants' families of origin.

Among the women who had experienced eating disorders, there were also
powerful themes about the significance of non-conditional relationships to
recovery (see Moulding, 2015). Carole, who described rape and emotional abuse
at the hands of her first husband as triggering her bulimia, went on to later talk
about her relationship with her current husband as an important part of her full
recovery: she said, 'he's the only person that has ever really loved me for just
being me, faults and all. There's no conditions, he accepts me'. Jade elaborated
on how her current boyfriend's love as well as relationships with 'people that
actually mattered' to her enabled her to 'just be completely me' rather than seek
social acceptance and belonging through thinness:

> Being with someone who loved me so much, I suppose that also helped
> because I felt I could just be completely me and that was like a wake-up
> call, you can still be you and feel loved. I think it just starting to feel com-
> fortable with myself like, as I got older I was getting to know myself and
> feeling more confident and caring less about what other people think. Yeah,
> just getting a better sense of who I am and stronger relationships with people
> that actually mattered to me as well.
>
> (Jade)

In line with humanist discourses of self-actualisation, Jade emphasised discovering and accepting her 'real' or 'true' self when she described 'getting a better
sense of who I am' (Lamoureux and Bortorff, 2005; Weaver *et al.*, 2005),
however, this was presented as part of being accepted unconditionally by others.
Thus, other studies emphasise the importance of unconditional relationships in
recovery from eating disorders (for example, Patching and Lawler, 2009), but
for the women in this study, these were often intertwined with, and enabled,
growing self-acceptance.

Falling off the merry-go-round

Some women who had left domestic violence talked about the importance of supportive relationships in moving on with their lives and overcoming the effects of violence and abuse. However, as noted, many women also talked about being actively isolated from other people in their lives through social abuse in domestic violence, with many violent men depicted as successfully blaming the women and turning family and friends against them. This could also include maternal alienation, where the women's own children were manipulated into taking their violent father's side against their mothers. Many women therefore talked about significant and seemingly permanent changes to their social and familial relationships as a result of gendered violence and coercive control. Of the women answering the open-ended survey question about emotional wellbeing, a full one-quarter (n = 139, 25 per cent) specifically mentioned, unprompted, that they no longer trusted other people because of domestic violence. Many specifically emphasised lack of trust in men and unwillingness to have another intimate relationship, but also lack of trust in others more generally and their reduced social networks and social isolation. Previous studies have also identified loss of trust in others as a result of domestic violence (for example, Scheffer Lindgren and Renck, 2008).

Women talked about the impact of domestic violence and coercive control on their other relationships in four main interrelated ways: their experiences of betrayal and lost trust in others; a lack of understanding of violence and abuse on the part of family and friends; withdrawal from others because of shame; and, a retreat on the part of many women into smaller worlds of safety, security and trust. Many women talked of feeling betrayed when friends or family sided with their partners during or after the violence and a resulting lack of trust in people. Jodie said that 'friends who supported me when I left the relationship don't talk to me'. Sometimes women suggested that this was a result of manipulation by partners as part of coercive control, for example, Tiffany said:

> I find it difficult to trust people such as family and friends as during the DV my ex turned my parents against me and my sister also. I won't allow myself to get close to friends.... I can't enjoy my life like I should because I am always safe-guarding myself from hurt.
>
> (Tiffany)

Tiffany talked about withdrawing from people in her life in order to safeguard herself from further hurt. Many other women talked about similar experiences of people turning away from them because of violence and abuse. Trista said:

> The truth of the situation [is that domestic violence] broke every friendship and family relationship I had and I lost my two best friends, three brothers completely and all others have been strained since from that time. I don't discuss the domestic violence with new people and have been isolated

socially being a single woman, everyone is partnered – I have not been to dinner at anyone's home for ten years, no catch ups in the evening with couples, just coffees with other school mums. I have been incredibly lonely.

(Trista)

Miranda also described no longer feeling trust in people, leading her to withdraw socially:

[I am] distrusting of people – men – lost faith in people, [I] do not feel comfortable entering into another relationship. [My] confidence and self-esteem were eroded. Some family members and friends turned away adding insult to an excruciatingly painful experience.

(Miranda)

Kaye said 'I can't trust anyone anymore. I feel people want to use me and hurt me like I'm just a joke', alluding to feelings of shame and humiliation. A little differently to some of the other women, Lizzie described her relationships with others in her life as damaged by the violence because she avoided friendships and withdrew from friends and family not wanting people 'to think that is you', implying feelings of shame about being seen as a victim of violence, and resulting social withdrawal and isolation. Marilyn not dissimilarly said, 'when you are in a mental and physically abusive relationship you keep it quiet because you are embarrassed'. Scheffer Lindgren and Renck (2008) also found that women feel high levels of shame and guilt, which can lead them to withdraw from others. Many women also blame themselves for the violence, in part because their partners used blame as part of domestic violence and to justify their violence (Scheffer Lindgren and Renck, 2008). Self-blame was common among the women in this study and shame about violence and abuse also acted as a barrier for some to developing or restoring a positive sense of themselves. However, Sara also drew attention to the class dimensions of this when she said 'I feel I have no self-worth. I feel empty. I feel that I have lost my old self. I feel dirty and lower class to my peers'. As shown in the previous chapter, many women suffer a significant drop in income, housing and employment status, with many sinking into poverty, and this and other accounts point to the shame and stigma that can be involved in this change of identity and the negative impact on social relationships.

Some of the women also talked about the fact that the people in their lives had difficulty grasping and understanding domestic violence, especially the more hidden forms of coercive control that occur out of public sight. For example, Emma said, 'normal people don't understand'. Winona described how difficult it was to get a close friend to understand her husband's behaviour because it did not accord with her own experience of him. This difference between the man the world sees and the man the woman knows was commonly referred to in the survey and interviews, with Elise saying how 'my ex-husband looked like a nice guy to everyone but behind the closed doors he would be a Jekyll and Hyde'. It is well-known that violent, controlling men carefully present a quite different façade to the wider world (Stark, 2007), and this can make it difficult for a woman to gain support because people cannot equate the woman's stories with the man they think they know. Gertrude similarly mentioned how neighbours could not believe her husband was violent and controlling because 'he was such a nice man outside the house. He was a devoted father and a devoted husband – but only if you did what he wanted to do'. Veronica's account offers a revealing counter to other women's experiences of not having their situations understood. She explained how her mother came to stay with her and saw for herself, first-hand, her partner's controlling and abusive behaviour. She said:

> She was really gobsmacked and so I could tell her look, I could ring her and just, I could tell her that I had a plan and then the plan would take eight months but I told her because I think it's very hard for people who are not in there to understand how you can still be with that person, why don't you just kick him out or isn't that just usual arguing, people don't really understand until they see it.
>
> (Veronica)

Veronica's mother provided critically important support that helped her leave safely because she understood from first-hand experience the nature of the behaviour her daughter was dealing with. However, the fact that violence and coercive control occur largely out of sight, behind closed doors, and men generally make sure no one sees it, makes it difficult for many women to gain this kind of support. Penny referred to having 'fallen off the merry-go-round' because of lost social connections and sense of self, as if she is no longer in the mainstream swim of life but outside it. Emilia explained that, because of her experiences of people not understanding and the danger this can bring should her ex-partner try and find her, she restricts her social life to those who have had similar experiences:

> I only invest in people who understand domestic violence and single motherhood and poverty ... my network is reliable, and empathic. I have no friends who have not experienced DV ... they often betray confidence and do not realise how dangerous the perpetrator is.... I am untrusting of other people.
>
> (Emilia)

Quantitative data from the survey shows that large numbers of women reported changes in their social and community activities during and after domestic violence in comparison to before violence. Many women reported decreases in friendship networks, contact with social groups and church groups during and after domestic violence. Many women also reported increases in contact with support groups (including domestic violence support groups) and political groups after domestic violence. These differences in social participation before, during and after domestic violence were statistically significant. Thus, many women's social worlds changed after domestic violence, with less contact with friends and social groups. While some of this change post-violence may be in part for reasons of safety, many women also mentioned experiences of betrayal, feeling that people do not understand and a resulting loss of trust in others. Such experiences are likely to contribute to poor mental health and the related lost sense of self and identity outlined in Chapter 7: as noted, social relationships are critical to identity and a sense of belonging is crucially important to quality of life and mental health and wellbeing (Bland *et al.*, 2015). I now move on to consider the implications for feminist-informed practice of women's narratives and experiences of helping-seeking, recovery and social relationships after gendered abuse.

Feminist practice

Feminist practitioners have a long history in responding to the consequences of gendered violence and abuse in women's lives, and here I draw on some of this repository of accumulated knowledge about feminist-informed practice in this area. Because this book has a focus on women's mental health, I focus on this area of intevention rather than other related areas such as child protection (see Itzin *et al.*, 2010 and Warner, 2009 for excellent discussions of feminist-informed child protection approaches). While there are many quality models for feminist-informed therapeutic work, I will touch on two here that seem to particularly resonate with many of the issues raised in this book. I also acknowledge that therapeutic approaches will differ according to the type of abuse experienced by women and the different types of mental health problems they face. However, I also want to attend to intervention beyond the individual in the spirit of attending to the discursive and material dimensions of women's experiences. As part of this, I draw on Nancy Tuana's (2006) concept of 'epistemologies of ignorance' to draw attention to the need to challenge community denial and resistance to knowledge about gendered violence and abuse. Tuana's (2006) idea of epistemologies of ignorance has been used by Franzway *et al.* (2009) in their examination of the sexual politics surrounding the under-representation of women in engineering. Franzway has more recently applied Tuana's concept to community denial about domestic violence. I argue that denial works to prevent meaningful responses to gendered violence, abuse and mental health, including both educational and structural action to reduce and prevent it into the future. I also argue that community denial worsens the mental health of women who have experienced gendered violence and abuse because it denies their lived reality.

Individual therapy with women

While two important approaches to feminist therapy with women who have experienced gendered violence and abuse are considered here, to reiterate, this is done in the knowledge that it is the quality of the relationship and rapport, empathy and understanding that are likely to be the most important dimensions in helping and supporting women. However, there are also important opportunities for situating women's distress in its gendered social context through feminist-informed therapy. The feminist-informed therapeutic approaches foregrounded here include narrative therapy and visible therapy. However, I acknowledge that there are many other approaches that will also have relevance and utility, and that practitioners often use a combination that can include traditional therapeutic techniques, such as cognitive-behavioural therapy, which can be effective for addressing specific symptoms of anxiety in particular, such as panic attacks.

Narrative therapy is not new and is now widely known and practised, so I will only briefly describe its approach. Narrative therapy is based on the work of White and Epston (1989), and has been widely used by social workers and other practitioners often, but not exclusively, based in non-traditional health care settings. White and Epston (1989) utilise the idea of 'stories' or 'narratives' around which individuals organise their lives, that give meaning to their experiences and through which they interact with others. People are understood to experience problems and seek help 'when the narratives in which they are "storying" their experience ... do not sufficiently represent their lived experience' because much of it contradicts the 'dominant narratives' (White and Epston, 1989: 22). White and Epston (1989) draw on the Foucauldian concept of power as productive, as inseparably tied up with knowledge and as producing truth. In particular, they adopt the Foucauldian idea of the normalising judgement of modern power to explain individuals' engagement in their own subjugation (White and Epston, 1989). They also utilise the idea of 'subjugated knowledges' that are 'exiled from the legitimate domain of the formal knowledges' whose 'insurrection' can provides a platform for resistance to dominant discourses and their power/knowledge effects (White and Epston, 1989: 30–31). These ideas are brought to the therapeutic 'conversation' by encouraging individuals in the identification of the 'truth discourses' that are subjugating them, and by 'resurrecting the subjugated knowledges' about the person and instances where they have resisted subjugation (White and Epston, 1989: 34). One of the key techniques for achieving this is externalisation (White and Epston, 1989). The technique of speaking about the problem – for example, 'abuse' or 'anxiety' – as it is an external entity is carried over into actual therapeutic conversations to challenge the idea of the person as the problem (see White and Epston, 1989; White, 1992). Michael White has described using a narrative therapy approach with a host of different problems faced by individuals, including working with those who have experienced trauma (White, 2004).

In a paper based on a presentation Michael White gave to the Treatment and Rehabilitation Center for Victims of Torture and Trauma in Ramallah, Palestine, he documents his narrative therapy approach with clients who have experienced trauma. White (2004) gives a fascinating account of how he used the techniques of 'double storied conversations' and 'doubly listening', and 'outsider witnessing'. He argues that his trauma work always involved 'double storied conversations' with the story about the trauma and the story about the response to trauma.

He describes 'doubly listening' as providing the opportunity for people to talk about what they might not have spoken about before, and listening for what they have continued to value in spite of trauma and their response to trauma. White (2004) also explains his use of 'outsider witnessing' in the case of trauma as providing an audience, often known to the client, for what the person gives value to based on the understanding that this has often been demeaned or disqualified as part of abuse, and that there can be little sense of a 'sense of myself' or agency for individuals with these experiences. I draw on the account of his work with one of the clients, 'Julie', who had experienced multiple traumas and a diagnosis of 'borderline personality disorder'. White explains that 'Julie' indicated

> no trace of that 'sense of myself' that is critical to the development of personal agency, to the development of an experience of the continuity of precious themes through the history, present and future of one's life, and to the development of intimate relationships with others.
>
> (2004: 53)

White (2004) identifies feelings of 'desolation, emptiness, incompetence, and worthlessness', as well as shame, as dominant responses to trauma for 'Julie' (p. 53). He credits naming what she valued in life in the context of 'a strongly resonant response through outsider-witnessing retellings' with the beginning of the process of reinvigorating 'Julie's' 'sense of myself'. Thus, outsider witnessing is understood and used to project images of identity for the client; the demonstration of an 'embodied interest' in the client through witnesses identifying their own reactions; and an acknowledgement of catharsis, which is taken to mean not only an emotional reaction to the client but the impact of the client's story in terms of witnesses' understandings of their own lives (White, 2004). As such, outsider witnessing is presented as positioning the person-in-relationship as an integral part of healing.

Clearly, the narrative approach to trauma is markedly different from psycho-medical approaches, with its embrace of post-structural ideas of the production of subjectivity in language, an embrace of the concept of multiple and fluid identities and the use of witnesses to enable the development of new senses of self in relationship with others. Interestingly, in the account above, White (2004) retains concepts that have their roots in humanist discourses of selfhood, such as a 'sense of myself' and the idea that a continuous sense of this through history is crucial to personal agency. Warner's (2009) visible therapy, based on a post-structural feminist perspective, takes a much more fluid approach to subjectivities. Warner (2009) describes her model as 'a critical, social and recovery oriented therapeutic approach to working with women and girls who have experienced child sexual abuse', involving a re-working of psychoanalytic theories through feminist and post-structural theories (p. 165). While Warner's (2009) visible therapy has been specifically developed to work with women and girls who have been sexually abused, it is possible that it could also be extended and adapted to other forms of gendered violence and abuse experienced by women. The aim of visible therapy is 'to challenge abuser-constructed reality by exploring how the tactics of abuse determine how women and girls come to understand themselves and their relationships in the world' (p. 165). Warner (2009) is particularly passionate about the need for therapy and therapeutic relationships to be transparent as a corrective to the client's earlier experiences of abusive relationships, which obscure how power operates to structure unequal, exploitative sexual relationships. Thus, the therapeutic relationship is conceived of as providing the alternative experience of a relationship based on partnership and democracy. In addition, and in line with a recovery approach, the therapist holds and communicates hope about the future to clients (Warner, 2009). The psychoanalytic concepts that are re-worked in visible therapy include the idea of defence mechanisms as coping strategies and challenging the assumption of 'healthy' heterosexual relationships as the measure of women's recoveries. Visible therapy also shares with narrative therapy a focus on the productive effects of language. However, Warner (2009) is also critical of aspects of narrative therapy, arguing that its 'extreme democratisation' can make therapists 'small' by denying their knowledge about abuse and its effects, which can have the inadvertent effect of reproducing abuse tactics of manipulation. Like narrative therapy, though, she encourages clients to explore multiple meanings of 'identities in relationship': this, she argues, 'allows clients and therapists to make sense of the ways power is transacted in relationships' (Warner, 2009: 174). However, this is arguably taken further than in White's (2004) description of working with clients with backgrounds of trauma. Warner (2009) argues that by focusing on small acts of control on the part of women, the 'felt sense of self can start to feel less stable and more constructed', working out which versions of self work in which situations (Warner, 2009: 176), contrasting with White's (2004) argument that a continuous sense of self is integral to personal agency. Nonetheless, both approaches offer thoughtful, highly ethical and progressive ways of working with women who have experienced gendered violence and abuse that challenge dominant psycho-medical approaches and their pathologising tendencies. These approaches also involve practitioners approaching the relationships in women's lives as inherently socio-political, rather than simply personal and individual, as part of supporting women in recognising gendered forms of social control in abuse.

Building trust, working through abuse and letting go are important stages of healing for all women who have experienced violence and abuse (Iztin *et al.*, 2010). Iztin *et al.* (2010) also talk about addressing the gendered nature of violence and abuse as part of working with women, such as the social construction of masculinities and the exertion of power and control over women by heterosexual men in intimate relationships. They also specifically highlight the importance of screening for gendered violence and abuse, and early intervention, particularly in health services where assumptions that domestic violence is a 'social problem' can lead to an unwillingness to enquire about women's experiences (Itzin *et al.*, 2010). They suggest that health workers need training in how to work with women who are or have been in domestic violence and are struggling with mental health issues. However, working with women who have experienced domestic violence also necessitates attending to safety and to the material conditions of women's lives by focusing on practical needs as well as the emotional distress wrought by violence and coercive control. This should also include attending to women's needs for social support networks. As noted earlier, the research conducted by my colleagues and myself, as well as that of other feminist researchers around the world, shows that domestic violence has a major long-term impact across many dimensions of women's lives. This perhaps draws attention most forcefully to the need for prevention and social change in relation to gendered violence and abuse.

Challenging community denial

Throughout the research presented in this book, women time and again referred to having their abuse silenced, ignored, denied or, at worst, being blamed for it themselves. Arguably, this was a major contributor to their mental health struggles beyond the traumatising experience of the abuse itself. As noted earlier in women's narratives of domestic violence in particular, the women not only described others failing to recognise or understand that they were experiencing gendered violence and coercive control, but also themselves prior to their first-hand experiences of it. In relation to childhood emotional abuse, many individuals talked about not realising that what they experienced was problematic until they visited friends' houses and saw that not everyone lived with high levels of conflict, violence and verbal abuse. Some described helping professionals failing or refusing to see any connections between their experiences of abuse and their experiences of mental illness. More specifically, a number of women described having their experiences of sexual abuse actively denied in families, or of being overtly blamed and held accountable for rape. In developing the concept of 'epistemologies of ignorance', Tuana (2006) argues that:

> to fully understand the complex practices of knowledge production and the variety of factors that account for why something is known, we must also understand the practices that account for *not* knowing, that is, for our *lack* of knowledge about a phenomenon.
>
> (Tuana, 2006: 2)

As is argued by Tuana (2006), 'understanding the various manifestations of ignorance and how they intersect with power requires attention to the permutations of ignorance in its different contexts' (p. 3). Through her examination of the women's health movement in the United States and its efforts to transform knowledge about women's bodies and health, Tuana (2006) offers a 'taxonomy of ignorance', elements of which have relevance to understanding ignorance and denial about gendered violence and abuse. Among the different types of ignorance, Tuana (2006) identifies wilful ignorance, which involves active ignoring of phenomena known to exist. This, she argues, describes the historical ignoring and denial of intra-familial child sexual abuse, which persists to this day in spite of feminist and professional efforts to challenge it. Arguably, wilful ignorance also extends to childhood emotional abuse, which has been know about for a long time but has received little formal, dedicated mainstream attention until recently. Tuana's (2006) concept of wilful ignorance is particularly relevant to the misunderstanding, denial and victim-blaming that surrounds domestic violence. As noted, in spite of widespread and regular reports about gendered violence in the media and from women's organisations, when individual women find themselves in such a situation, they and the people around them do not necessarily recognise and identify it as such.

However, knowing about the *gendered* nature of violence and abuse arguably also suffers from another form of ignorance, which Tuana (2006) describes as '*not knowing that we do not know*' (p. 6). This type of ignorance stems from the fact that current interests, beliefs and theories in society work to obscure certain forms of knowledge (Tuana, 2006). The current interests and beliefs that are relevant to 'not knowing' about the gendered dimensions of violence and abuse, and their impact on women's mental health, include the dominance of positivist science in medicine and psychology and its adherence to 'objectivity' and supposed gender neutrality, as well as arguments about 'gender symmetry' in domestic violence. As have shown throughout this book, this so-called gender-neutral stance is in fact gender-blind and works to obscure the operation of gender and gender power relations in violence abuse, including its differential impact on women and men. Dominant contemporary discourses about gender equality are also relevant to 'not knowing' about the gendered dimensions of violence and abuse, and their impact on mental health. These promulgate the idea that women and men are now equal and often embrace the concomitant (and usually unstated) belief that it is therefore 'sexist' to explore the possibility that women's and men's experiences might in fact differ in important ways that have little to do with supposed 'natural' gender differences. Thus, discourses and assumptions about gender equality described in Chapter 6 can cloud and obscure the *unequal* social conditions so fundamental to gendered violence and coercive control. Tuana (2006) also argues that some 'knowers' are epistemically disadvantaged because:

> cognitive authority is determined by many factors, including the character of a speaker, her or his intellectual capacity, his or her reasonableness, and so on – criteria that feminists have demonstrated to be imbued with the prejudices of sexism, androcentrism, racism, classism, ageism, and ableism.
>
> (Tuana, 2006: 13)

Being a woman in and of itself is likely to bring assumptions of greater emotionality, irrationality and therefore reduced credibility (Ussher, 2010), and women (and children) are likely to be particularly psychologically distressed and fearful when they disclose experiences of gendered violence and abuse, reducing their credibility further. Further to this, though, as pointed out in previous chapters, numerous discourses that actively blame women and girls for the abuse they experience are in circulation in this area that arguably reduce even further their credibility as authoritative knowers about violence and abuse. In relation to domestic violence, women paint a picture of their partners that is at odds with many people's experience and knowledge of him, and which is often actively contrived as such by controlling male partners: it is not difficult to see that he may be believed over her, or that at the very least she may be simply dismissed, especially if she has been cast as mentally unstable. Men who abuse children are also known to be adept at painting a quite different picture of themselves outside the home (Herman, 2000), while abusive parents can commonly blame the child for their own abusive behaviour. Thus, this disjuncture between how others see perpetrators of abuse, and the victim's version, can work to reduce women's (and children's) credibility as reporters of violence and abuse. Other gendered discourses that position women as responsible for relationships and for creating a happy home and family also further enable victim-blaming and wilful ignorance (Moulding *et al.*, 2015). Most importantly, though, proper recognition of gendered violence and abuse requires acceptance that widespread gender inequalities persist, and that as long as this knowledge continues to be resisted, the wilful ignorance of 'knowing that we know but don't want to know' will persist and action to properly address and redress gendered violence and abuse will be avoided. More specifically, I argue that epistemologies of ignorance about gendered violence and abuse contribute to women's ongoing struggles with sense of self, identity and belonging, helping to undermine their emotional wellbeing beyond the immediate effects of gendered violence and abuse itself.

Community denial of gendered violence and abuse draws attention to the need for societal attitudinal change – symbolic change – about women, men, violence and male privilege. This also needs to extend to non-pathologising understandings of mental health problems that situates them in their social and gendered contexts. There are efforts at both the national and international levels by governments across the world to challenge community denial and increase awareness of gendered violence and abuse, for example, through UN Women and the National Plan to Reduce Violence against Women and their Children 2010–2022 adopted by the Australian federal government in 2013. At both national and international levels, prevention is also understood as necessitating structural change through the promotion of gender equality. As has been well-established in the public health field, change is not possible without a coordinated effort that includes both educational and structural interventions (Itzin *et al.*, 2010). In redressing gendered violence and abuse, improving mental health services to women (Itzin *et al.*, 2010), support services to women and children and improving criminal justice responses are also critical (Australian Council of Health Ministers, 2013). While international and national policy statements are undoubtedly positive steps that include many vital elements, they require ongoing commitments from governments, which are often more focused on, and concerned with, reducing spending. As noted earlier, violence against women has become a pivotal battleground for the contemporary women's movement across the world. More than anything else, I argue that galvanising and reinvigorating the feminist movement around violence against women perhaps offers the most important challenge to the community denial and gender inequalities that produce and reproduce gendered violence and the mental health problems that arise in response to it.

References

Anthony, W.A. (1993) Recovery from mental illness: the guiding vision of the mental health service system in the 1990s. *Psychosocial Rehabilitation Journal*, 16(4), pp. 11–23.

Australian Bureau of Statistics (ABS) (2007) *National Mental Health and Wellbeing Survey*. Canberra.

Australian Council of Health Ministers (2013) *National Plan to Reduce Violence against Women and their Children 2010–2022*. Canberra.

Bjork, T. and Ahlstrom, G. (2008) The patient's perception of having recovered from an eating disorder. *Health Care for Women International*, 29(8–9), pp. 926–944.

Bland, R., Renouf, N. and Tullgren, A. (2015) *Social Work Practice in Mental Health: An Introduction*. Crows Nest: Allen & Unwin.

Davidson, L., O'Connell, M.J., Tondora, J., Lawless, M. and Evans, A.C. (2005) Recovery in serious mental illness: a new wine or just a new bottle?, *Professional Psychology: Research and Practice*, 36(5), pp. 480–487.

Deegan, P. (1996) Recovery as a journey of the heart. *Psychiatric Rehabilitation Journal*, 19(3), pp. 91–97.

Doyle, C. (2001) Surviving and coping with emotional abuse in childhood, *Clinical Child Psychology and Psychiatry*, 6(3), pp. 387–402.

Frank, A.W. (1995) *The Wounded Storyteller: Body, Illness, and Ethics*. Chicago: University of Chicago Press.

Franzway, S., Sharp, R., Mills, J.E. and Gill, J. (2009) Engineering ignorance: the problem of gender equity in engineering, *Frontiers*, 30(1), pp. 89–106.

Garrett, C. (1998) *Beyond Anorexia: Narrative, Spirituality and Recovery*. Cambridge: Cambridge University Press.

Hajjar, L. (2004) Religion, state power, and domestic violence in Muslim societies: a framework for comparative analysis, *Law and Social Inquiry*, 29(1), pp. 1–38.

Herman, J.L. (2000) *Father-Daughter Incest*. Cambridge, MA: Harvard University Press.

Humphreys, C. and Thiara, R. (2003) Mental health and domestic violence: 'I call it symptoms of abuse', *British Journal of Social Work*, 33(2), pp. 209–226.

Itzin, C., Taket, A. and Barter-Godfrey, S. (2010) *Domestic and Sexual Violence and Abuse: Tackling the Health and Mental Health Effects*. Abingdon: Routledge.

Lamoureux, M.M.H. and Bottorff, J.L. (2005) 'Becoming the real me': recovering from anorexia nervosa, *Health Care for Women International*, 26(2), pp. 170–188.

McAdams, D.P., Reynolds, J., Lewis, M., Patten, A.H. and Bowman, P.J. (2001) When bad things turn good and good things turn bad: sequences of redemption and contamination in life narrative and their relation to psychosocial adaptation in midlife adults and in students. *Personality and Social Psychology Bulletin*, 27, pp. 472–483.

Moulding, N.T. (2015) Gendered intersubjectivities in narratives of recovery from an eating disorder, *Affilia: The Journal of Women in Social Work*, first published online 16 March 2015, doi:10.1177/0886109915576519.

Moulding, N.T., Buchanan, F. and Wendt, S. (2015) Untangling self-blame and mother-blame in women's and children's perspectives on maternal protectiveness in domestic violence: implications for practice, *Child Abuse Review*, published online 12 May 2015, DOI: 10.1002/car.2389.

Patching, J. and Lawler, J. (2009) Understanding women's experiences of developing an eating disorder and recovering: a life-history approach, *Nursing Inquiry*, 16(1), pp. 10–21.

Scheffer Lindgren, M.S. and Renck, B. (2008) 'It is still so deep-seated, the fear': psychological stress reactions as consequences of intimate partner violence, *Journal of Psychiatric and Mental Health Nursing*, 15(3), pp. 219–228.

Stark, E. (2007) *Coercive Control: How Men Trap Women in Personal Life*. Oxford: Oxford University Press.

Thomas, S.P. and Hall, J.M. (2008) Life trajectories of female child abuse survivors thriving in adulthood, *Qualitative Health Research*, 18, pp. 149–166.

Tuana, N. (2006) The speculum of ignorance: the women's health movement and epistemologies of ignorance, *Hypatia*, 21(3), pp. 1–19.

Ussher, J. (2010) Are we medicalizing women's misery: a critical review of women's higher rates of reported depression, *Feminism and Psychology*, 20(9), pp. 9–35.

Warner, S. (2009) *Understanding the Effects of Child Sexual Abuse: Feminist Revolutions in Theory, Research and Practice*. London: Routledge.

Weaver, K., Wuest, J. and Ciliska, D. (2005) Understanding women's journey of recovering from anorexia nervosa, *Qualitative Health Research*, 15, pp. 188–206.

White, M. (1992) Deconstruction and therapy. In D. Epston and M. White (eds), *Experience, Contradiction, Narrative and Imagination: Selected Papers of David Epston and Michael White, 1989–1991*. Adelaide: Dulwich Centre Publications.

White, M. (2004) Working with people who are suffering the consequences of multiple trauma: a narrative perspective, *The International Journal of Narrative Therapy and Community Work*, 1, pp. 44–75.

White, M. and Epston, D. (1989) *Literate Means to Therapeutic Ends*. Adelaide: Dulwich Centre Publications.

8   Final comments

Throughout this book, I have endeavoured to take an interconnected feminist approach to gendered violence, abuse and mental health by considering different types of abuse together, and exploring how they can play out in different kinds of emotional distress for women. I have also attempted to navigate both the discursive and material, lived dimensions of women's understandings and experiences simultaneously, in line with the concept of situated intersubjectivity (McNay, 2004). Among other things, what this approach has enabled is the identification of both the diversity of discourses framing women's experiences but also some broad themes that appear to be relatively common to women's experiences of mental health problems in response to gendered violence and abuse. In particular, all three studies draw attention to the way that contradictory discourses about femininity frame gendered violence and abuse, and also underpin psycho-medical discourses used to explain and treat the mental health problems women experience as a result of violence and abuse. At the basis of this lies persistent and gendered social contradictions about femininity and its problematic relation to personhood and selfhood in Western cultures, which other feminists examining gender and mental health have previously identified (for example, Bordo, 1993; MacSween, 1993; Wirth-Cauchon, 2001). Further to this, though, the analysis undertaken in this book illustrates how gendered violence and abuse exaggerates and amplifies these gender contradictions, causing significant emotional distress to women along the way that is then reified as 'mental illness', hiding the operation of the gender discourses and power relations framing these dynamics.

Exploration of childhood emotional abuse in Chapter 4 demonstrated that women's and men's narratives and experiences include significant gendered dimensions that have a number of implications for how the impact of abuse might be managed in individual lives. I showed how hegemonic masculinities (Connell, 2005) framed the men's narratives, constructing 'manhood' as a unitary and fundamentally good thing that was entirely commensurate with being a 'good person'. I also showed how this involved a centring of the control of emotion and sometimes a positioning of femininity as lesser. In contrast, the women talked about themselves in non-gendered terms while often depicting highly gendered practices of shaming, guilt, manipulation and control based on contradictory femininities that undermined personhood. I argued that these tensions and contradictions are experienced to some extent by all women, but can be dramatically brought to life in childhood emotional abuse to produce powerful feelings of worthlessness, anxiety, guilt, confusion, shame and a sense of not being able to win either way. The analysis also showed that while the women had access to other apparently gender-neutral discourses about themselves as autonomous persons, these are based on masculinist assumptions about personhood and autonomy that sit in some tension with femininity discourses (Burman, 1996). Thus, contradictory and subjugated femininities could leave women with the impression that there is something fundamentally wrong with *them*, which throws some light on the social processes framing so-called 'internalisation' of abuse-related emotion for women and its 'externalisation' for men. The analysis of women's and men's narratives and experiences of childhood emotional abuse therefore showed how they are framed by gendered social discourses and related practices that risk entrenching binaries of gender along relatively traditional lines.

The abuse depicted by some of the women in the eating disorder study also rested on highly conflicted discourses and related expectations about gender. Hence, some women described emotional and physical abuse focused on expectations they would be non-sexual, dependent and care for others against more contemporary invitations to autonomy and independence, while sexual abuse involved a contradictory positioning as both passive victim and as responsible for abuse. Conflicted discourses about femininity as living for others versus living for oneself therefore structured the women's narratives and experiences of abuse, and played out in their subsequent struggles over food and weight. Moreover, gendered forms of abuse magnified wider cultural ambivalences about femininity, producing powerful emotions such as shame that played out in the use of food as a similarly conflicted solution. I then showed how shame is a particularly gendered emotion (Probyn, 2005), with self-starvation and bingeing focused on relieving and overcoming such feelings.

Examination of women's narratives and experiences of domestic violence and mental health in Chapter 6 revealed women's ongoing fears about physical danger as well as the navigation of deep-seated, gendered contradictions for the women about who they are, their worth and their place in the world. Again, I showed how gendered violence and coercive control exaggerate the already existing gender contradictions in women's day-to-day lives about being at once subject and object, person and non-person. While all women face such contradictions to some extent, like other forms of gendered violence and abuse, domestic violence 'turns up the volume' and thereby turns up the associated emotional distress, which is also overlayed with fears of current physical and sexual violence. The narratives and experiences of women who have left domestic violence were also distinguished by the negative impact of domestic violence on the material conditions of many women's lives, such as income, housing and employment. These material impacts sometimes appeared to compound women's emotional distress and the dilemmas around sense of self and identity described by many of the women. Lastly, in all of the studies, women resisted the medicalisation of their distress. Indeed, anger emerged as one of the dominant 'structures of feeling' among the women who had left domestic violence, framed by contemporary discourses of individual rights and gender equality. However, some women also embraced the diagnosis of PTSD as an explanation for their distress because it is one of the only readily available discourses offered by psycho-medicine that draws attention to the social basis of their mental health experiences.

All three studies highlighted the emotional dimensions of gendered violence and abuse, with women commonly identifying feelings of shame, self-blame, guilt, worthlessness, sadness and fear as central to their emotional distress. However, these emotions were placed in their gendered social contexts as reflective of gender discourses, practices and power relations rather than signs of individual pathology. In exploring feminist-informed approaches to intervention, I considered some of the key principles and approaches to working with women who have experienced gendered violence, abuse and mental health problems, such as the importance of language in constructing identity, the idea of multiple identities rather than idealised masculinist notions of autonomy and the situating of women's emotional distress in the socio-political power relations and relationships in their lives (Warner, 2009; White, 2004). I also drew attention to White's (2004) observation that a stronger 'sense of myself' over time is important to personal agency, in addition to awareness of the socially contingent nature of identity. I agree that strengthening 'sense of self' can be particularly significant for women with backgrounds of violence and abuse because as these studies have shown, the undermining of feminine selfhood is so central to the tactics of gendered violence and abuse. In the spirit of attending to the symbolic, material and structural dimensions of gendered violence, abuse and mental health, I also pointed to the need for societal attitude change about women, 'mental illness', violence and male privilege as well as simultaneous efforts to reduce structural gender inequalities.

Over the period that I have been writing this book, violence against women has been increasingly gaining attention both here in Australia and around the world. While it is positive that the silence that has historically surrounded gendered violence and abuse is lifting once again, it is also important to be cognisant of the fact that this social problem has been repeatedly 'discovered' and then 'forgotten' in the face of denial, continuing male privilege and gender inequalities. The reduction of gendered violence and abuse against women and children is one of the most important social problems to be tackled over the next few decades, and it is therefore a critical time for a reinvigorated women's movement to be involved in forging safer living environments for women and children both inside and outside their homes.

References

Bordo, S. (1993) *Unbearable Weight: Feminism, Western Culture and the Body*. Berkeley: University of California Press.

Burman, E. (1996) The spec(tac)ular economy of difference. In S. Wilkinson and C. Kitzinger (eds), *Representing the Other*. London: Sage Publications, pp. 138–140.

Connell, R.W. (2005) *Masculinities*, second edition. Crows Nest: Allen & Unwin.

McNay, L. (2004) Situated intersubjectivity. In B. Marshall and A. Witz (eds), *Engendering the Social: Feminist Encounters with Sociological Theory*. Maidenhead: Open University Press, pp. 171–186.

MacSween, M. (1993) *Anorexic Bodies*. London: Routledge.

Probyn, E. (2005) *Blush: Faces of Shame*, Minneapolis: University of Minnesota Press.

Warner, S. (2009) *Understanding the Effects of Child Sexual Abuse: Feminist Revolutions in Theory, Research and Practice*. London: Routledge.

White, M. (2004) Working with people who are suffering the consequences of multiple trauma: a narrative perspective, *The International Journal of Narrative Therapy and Community Work*, 1, pp. 44–75.

Wirth-Cauchon, J. (2001) *Borderline Personality Disorder: Symptoms and Stories*. Piscataway: Rutgers University Press.

Index